That is Not Me

A Journey of Perception

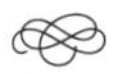

BY L.J. NELSON

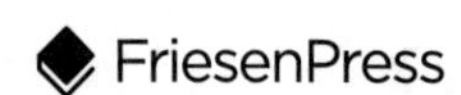

Suite 300 - 990 Fort St
Victoria, BC, V8V 3K2
Canada

www.friesenpress.com

First Edition — 2018

ISBN
978-1-5255-1973-4 (Hardcover)
978-1-5255-1974-1 (Paperback)
978-1-5255-1975-8 (eBook)

1. BIOGRAPHY & AUTOBIOGRAPHY, PEOPLE WITH DISABILITIES

Distributed to the trade by The Ingram Book Company

That Is Not Me: A Journey of Perception is dedicated to the memory of my parents, family, and friends who have passed.

To them and to those who have influenced me in this journey, thank you.

This book was written for all who are walking their own personal journeys of difference.

While the narrative is a reflection of my life, all names of persons, except my own, referred to in this book have been changed to protect their privacy.

L.J. Nelson

That is Not Me

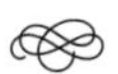

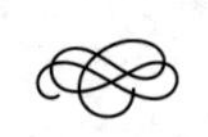

Introduction

The theme of my life's story is based on a poem that was, along with other poems, written more than thirty years ago. It was a time when I was driven to complete my educational training, become a competent professional, and hopefully be an independent, contributing participant of society. It was a time when I realized that my life, while "normal" in so many ways, has never been, nor would ever actually be, normal at all. It was a time when reality hit me with a force that cannot be described, and it has taken me over a quarter of a century to discover what my actual reality or perception of life is.

I remember one of the first times I was accused by an adult of lying. I was attending a Brownie troop meeting and as a nine-year-old was very terrified of our troop leader. She was a retired high school teacher who was greatly respected for her teaching career and achievements. She had an Old English presence about her and was very formal with her words. She had asked the Brownies to list in their groups the signs of spring, particularly naming different plants and fauna that give evidence of spring.

Anyone who is close to me knows that while I can appreciate nature, I have zero skills in labelling the scientific names of plants or animals. A bird is a bird, and a flower is a flower. I was so in need of contributing to the discussion that I named a flower I believed was in my mother's flower garden – a rose. The small group leaders were sharing their lists with the larger group. As the word 'rose' was read out, our troop leader loudly interrupted and wanted to know who had suggested a rose.

The battle was on. I did not back down. I was not going to admit I had no idea what that pink flower in my mother's flower garden was called. Instead, I was adamant that I had seen a rose. The same is true for the recollections of my life. In order for me to tell a story involving incidents that occurred so long ago, sometimes the tulip I am attempting to describe may be, in fact, a rose.

Perception is a twist of what reality is. Perception protects us from the truth. Perception can be handled, even manhandled, to suit our needs. The perception of my life's journey is just that, mine.

During the past fifteen years, I have experienced many unexpected challenges in this journey. From these challenges, new paths have been opened. I believe there are others who have walked a similar road. I also believe that sharing my story with others may help guide someone in their own journey.

My family and friends might view this journey from a little different perspective; however, none of them has actually walked in my shoes. This is my path.

The title of this book is a phrase I commonly reply with when strangers approach me and insist I am someone else. 'That Is Not Me,' a grammatically incorrect phrase that I have used repeatedly when trying to explain to those who assume I am someone I am not. This is an opportunity to share my story of me.

L.J. Nelson

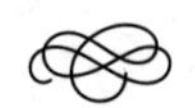

Life would be different if I was not me.
I would stand tall and be proud of who I am.
Instead, my life is wasted and I look back in pain.
The pain of my family, the selfishness and greed.
The pain of my friends, the comfort and lies.
The pain of a stranger, the names,
the eyes, the degradation.
The pain of the one I love,
the obsessive giving to one who does not see.
The pain of a kiss, of a dance or a hug,
these things I cannot miss since I've never known them.
The question of being normal will never be forgotten.

—L.J. Nelson, December 1983

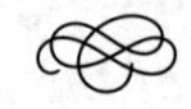

Chapter 1

Life would be different if I was not me

I was born in a small city hospital in Saskatchewan in the early 1960s. I weighed seven pounds, three ounces and was twenty-one inches long. The medical care professionals regarded this birth as normal and I was sent home after the mandatory three-day hospital stay. Soon afterwards, a nurse, who later became a great support for my family, approached my mother and informed her that the size of my head seemed unusually large. While uncertain what condition I had, this professional believed that something was wrong.

The diagnosis, when made three months later, was a mystery to the professionals in our community. I was given the diagnosis of achondroplasia, a form of dwarfism, medically known as skeletal dysplasia. There were only a few professionals in my province that knew what this condition meant. My family would experience a lot of ignorance, numerous prejudices and preconceived judgements of the condition for many years afterwards.

Dwarfism has never really been a well-known medical condition and even today, many medical professionals have limited understanding of the needs and particulars of persons who have any form of skeletal dysplasia. In the early 1960s, there were no substantial supports for families encountering dwarfism, particularly in Canada, and especially in Saskatchewan.

Dwarfism, unlike many other physical or motor disabilities, cannot readily be fixed or cured with a physical aid or rehabilitation. For people with achondroplasia, the most common form of dwarfism, a genetic mutation occurs that causes the skeleton, particularly the arms and legs, to grow in a different manner. With the increased emphasis on studies related to this genetic condition, many recent discoveries have been made about skeletal dysplasia disorders.

This increased interest in genetic research regarding the causes of achondroplasia has resulted in recent findings that, to a layperson, are quite complex in the terminology used in studies. A decade ago, it was determined that it was the male partner, who contributed the genetic mutation, which defined those with achondroplasia. The idea that this research, which has recently led to initial drug trials in the States, may someday stop the mutation of the cartilage as it is formed into bone before birth is something I had never entertained as possible.

Little People are different. Those with achondroplasia have a skull shape that is irregular and somewhat larger than normal. We walk with a waddling gait because of the placement of our hips and the reverse curvature of our spines. Our voices are of a higher pitch. Our facial features are distinctive and many of us experience secondary conditions such as sleep apnea and respiratory disorders because of the restrictions of our airways. Every bone in our body, particularly those within our limbs, is of a shape that is not within the norm.

Other forms of dwarfism have their own distinct growth patterns and mutations. The most similar form of dwarfism to achondroplasia is pseudoachondroplasia. The adult height range and body types are similar, yet we are different because of our facial features. The pseudo's facial characteristics seem more familiar within their own family's resemblance to the norm. Another form, diastrophic dwarfism, is a rarer type where those affected are somewhat shorter than "Achons" and experience ongoing spinal challenges because of their different growth patterns.

Simply, but by no means accurately, as a dwarf, the way our bones grow is different. The reason, or etiology, for our condition ranges from inheriting those traits from our parents who may also have dwarfism, to an unexplained genetic mutation with no evidence of previous conditions within the family tree. I am one of those unexplained cases.

There is an oxymoron within my condition. In the medical field, I am not considered disabled or unique. Being healthy as a Little Person means I do not qualify in Canada as having a physical disability. As an achondroplasia person ages, though, the degree of other secondary conditions becomes more apparent. There is stress upon certain organs as they become squished or as the wear and tear on our disfigured skeletal system reaches a critical point. My secondary symptoms can qualify for benefits and in recent years, I have benefitted from income tax credits.

How I was raised has been a great determiner of who I am today. I was the second youngest of seven children and, while we lived in a city in Saskatchewan, we were also a farm family. All of my siblings are of average height. My parents strived to create a "normal" environment for me as I was growing up. My mother became the expert on my condition. She was a teacher and viewed my challenges as lessons in life. My father was the nurturer of the family. His role for me was one of emotional support and stability. I was fortunate to have a blend of these two parental styles. My mother's view may seem harsh compared to current trends in raising children who are different, but I benefitted by becoming independent and productive as an adult.

I encountered numerous medical and physical challenges as a young infant. Within the first year of my life, I struggled through three bouts of pneumonia. While I was speaking quite fluently by the age of two, I did not start walking until I passed three years of age. Acquiring the proper type of footwear to encourage stability and balance was a constant challenge during my preschool years. It took many years for me to master the art of walking, and I ended up having a few significant spills while descending steps in our home.

While my medical file was quite thick, the majority of doctor visits during my early years were for the numerous examinations and studies to monitor my growth. Ongoing visits to various doctors to monitor my progress, particularly at the Royal University Hospital in Saskatoon, occurred. At one point, I recall actually being paid by this teaching hospital for a time to be a "real-life example" for interns and residents to study and examine.

Upon birth, every organ within our chest cavity is of the same size as an average person. The challenge is finding space for these organs to develop as we age. My medical challenges centred on my lungs' ability to fight off infections and on the common female reproductive issues that other women encounter in their twenties and thirties.

My parents became quite creative with some of the physical challenges I encountered as I was growing up. Our family home had two door handles on the front outside door. I had to wait for someone to answer my knock if the inside doors were closed. It took a few years, but I eventually developed skill in balancing on the lower ledge of the doorframe while at the same time manipulating the round inside doorknob.

As a young preschooler, I recall carrying a large purse around with me continually. It wasn't until my adolescent years that it was disclosed that this purse was filled with weights in an attempt to straighten my arms that would not fully extend. While I have complete rotation of my joints, my ability to extend my arms in a straight line is still not possible.

My lower limbs from the knee to my ankle are significantly bowed. Being bow-legged as a Little Person is very common for our generation since the therapies that are now readily available to prevent this condition were not known at the time. Occasionally, secondary conditions such as tight tendons and muscles, resulting from moving differently, have created further complications for people with dwarfism.

During the 1960s, the public had little knowledge of dwarfism and many people believed that this achondroplasia condition also involved limited cognitive functioning. With that assumption, when I reached the proper age to enter into my first year of schooling, officials attempted to convince my parents that the best placement for me would be in a segregated school designated for children with significantly lower cognitive functioning. For my parents, this recommendation was not going to be considered and definitely was not accepted. I was enrolled in our local public school and continued my education, completing a Bachelor of Education degree seventeen years later.

My memories of growing up seem to be the same as children in my neighbourhood. In fact, very few adaptations were actually provided in my home. I was expected to make meals and do various chores with little assistance or accommodations. The dishes and food items were stored on upper shelves. The pots were stored high above the stove. Daily, I had to climb to reach needed items. During my early years, we had step-stool chairs that we would use at the kitchen table, along with one metal step stool in our home that was stored behind the kitchen door.

Everything I did in the kitchen required some sort of vertical uprising. I thought nothing of pulling out a chair, climbing upon it and completing whatever task I needed to accomplish. An expectation for me, which I seemed to need constant reminding of, was to return the chairs and stools to their designated place when not in use.

To provide additional challenges, sometime in the mid-1970s, my parents purchased new kitchen furniture: an octagon table along with four swivel armchairs that would roll on wheels – very stylish at the time. The only thing I liked about these chairs were the padded arms that I could stand on to raise myself even higher while reaching. I can recall repeatedly standing on the arm of one of these wheeled chairs hoping it wouldn't roll away as I was searching for a dish.

To remove the wet, clingy laundry from the bottom of the top-loading washing machine, I used the handle end of a broom. The two large freezers in the basement, though, always seemed to be my nemesis. Standing on a chair or stool, I was still challenged by the distance to reach frozen items from the bottom of the freezer. It took me years to figure out, but eventually, I started using the flat blades of my brothers' hockey sticks that they had left lying in the basement.

The differences in the way I completed tasks were common practices for me and it never occurred to me that others might view this as abnormal. Many who were unfamiliar with my ability to move or transport weighty items thought nothing of grabbing items from me before inquiring if I needed help. My family knew me and understood why it was important to complete tasks on my own. Even today, a stranger watching me walk along a counter top in a kitchen cannot help but want to intervene and offer assistance, thinking I am at risk.

Some may have viewed my parents as lacking in regard for my physical needs, or possibly some would even see this as parental neglect. Not so; I feel that everything they didn't do to rescue me was purposeful. I developed lifelong skills in being able to identify a problem, creatively formulate solutions, and most especially, I developed a strong sense of order and need for independence. My parents didn't rescue me from those daily challenges; they headed me straight into them. I was expected to drive, so I drove. I was expected to work, so I worked. There were not long discussions or formulated plans for achieving success with tasks. There was just a constant expectation that I would succeed.

My need for independence as I developed into a teenager was extremely important for me and I couldn't wait until I was old enough to drive a car. That was my ultimate independence goal and continues to be a necessity of life. My parents started talking about different choices for modifying a vehicle a few years before I was of age. I started the driver education course at high school along with my classmates of similar age. There were no problems with the written work; however, I did encounter some challenges during the training.

In those days, you were required to complete so many hours on a simulator prior to practicing driving in a car. My scores from the computer program were dismal each time. I had great scores for required steering and signalling, but repeated failures for the acceleration and braking skills. My feet couldn't reach the pedals.

The in-vehicle practice lessons were also not possible. While the driver education car was outfitted with dual controls for the instructor to intervene if necessary, there were no accommodations such as raised pedals or a hand control for me. It was at this time that my parents were discussing the modifications needed on our vehicle for me. I would need a raised seat and a hand control installed.

Fortunately for me, and unfortunately for my middle brother who was involved, our existing vehicle was totalled in an accident. This required purchasing a new car and the car purchased had electric seats. Cool, very cool. I now wouldn't have to sit on foam pillows to see above the steering wheel.

My driver education teacher was an enjoyable man who didn't panic while teaching adolescents how to drive, at least up until it was time to teach me. When teaching most students, he had his own steering wheel and brakes in his car, but not in mine. Our new vehicle had arrived and the local dealership had installed the hand control. We were set for driving.

The first lesson was driving in an empty parking lot at the mall but I soon advanced to busier roadways and streets. Since there had already been a delay in acquiring a new vehicle for our family and I had already passed my sixteenth birthday, I wanted to complete as many lessons as possible, as fast as possible, in order to drive. It was a month later that I acquired my real independence and passed the road test. I always believed that disallowing the driver examiner the same needed permission that the driver instructor asked about draping his leg across the console to access the brake influenced the outcome of the examination.

They say that driving is a privilege and a reward. For me, driving is my gift. I know that someday when I am older I will be challenged with the idea of sustaining that privilege, but right now, it is a vital part of me. I have continued to use a hand control for driving even though access to alternative adaptations such as pedal extenders are now available.

As an adult, I have different accommodations throughout my home and workplace to assist my needs. The availability of appliances such as refrigerators with side-by-side doors, front-loading washing machines and microwave drawers have made a positive difference for me. Lever door handles and lower standard height for light switches have been helpful. Foldable one-step plastic stools are now a common purchase item and can be taken everywhere.

While some adjustments and accommodations can be easily made with little expense, repetitive climbing and carrying stools to reach everything above the height of a kitchen counter is impractical and takes a toll on one's body over the years. I have been fortunate to have the means to own my own home and have had extensive custom renovations completed to suit those needs over time. The most recent change involved renovating the entire upper floor including custom cupboards in my kitchen. The acquisition of a kitchen island built at my height allows me to prepare meals and clean up my workspace without ever climbing onto a stool or chair.

We become accustomed to what we have, and for me to adapt to the average person's living space was done without thinking. I lived and worked in places where people of average height lived. There were exceptions, though. I was fortunate in my workplace to be primarily working with younger children and so had access to child-height chairs and tables. The need for adaptations in my home and in my workplace increased as I aged when I started finding the repetitive climbing tasks more physically challenging. If it were not for my secondary condition with my spine, I would probably have continued using chairs and stools to reach high objects without thinking twice about the additional physical effort involved.

Seeking different perspectives and finding my own solutions was in large part due to the manner in which I was raised. Today, families of Little People have access to abundant knowledge, support and, at times, the financial means of providing physical accommodations for their children in their homes as they are growing up. There is a risk, though, in providing too many accommodations for children who are vertically challenged. If that child grows up in an environment where all their challenges are accommodated, they will become accustomed to having their comforts always provided and will not experience those personal achievements and opportunities to find their own solutions. The opposite is also true. For families with limited knowledge or means of providing for their children who have dwarfism, their primary goal becomes a need to protect them from the harsh, sometimes cruel world of society. That person's world becomes very restrictive and they become dependent upon those close to them. In a way, they are protected from the hurt or disappointment that may come their way, but they are also hidden from life.

From my view, I believe there needs to be a balance between the provision of supports, as well as encouraging the expectation of independence. An individual's needs are personal to their particular physical challenges, their understandings, and life experiences. Building design and structures are better suited for short-statured people. The majority of our world, though, continues to be designed for those who are average in height.

I can scream loudly and insist that all public venues be accessible to me. I have screamed at times when facilities are decades behind the current laws of inclusive access, such as out-of-reach elevator buttons. However, to scream every time I come across something that I cannot access or obtain because of my height would mean constantly screaming in a world that is bigger than I am.

The me I am today is because of the difference in the way I was raised. If I had been raised in an environment of complete accommodation and expectation that every challenge encountered would be solved for me, then yes, life would be different if I was not me. If I had been raised in an over-protective bubble where I was provided for, but not encouraged to interact with others or explore the possibilities of this world, then yes, life would be different if I was not me. Instead, I'm thankful for the manner in which I was raised and that I continue to have opportunities of vertical challenges because life is different because I am me.

Life is different because I am me

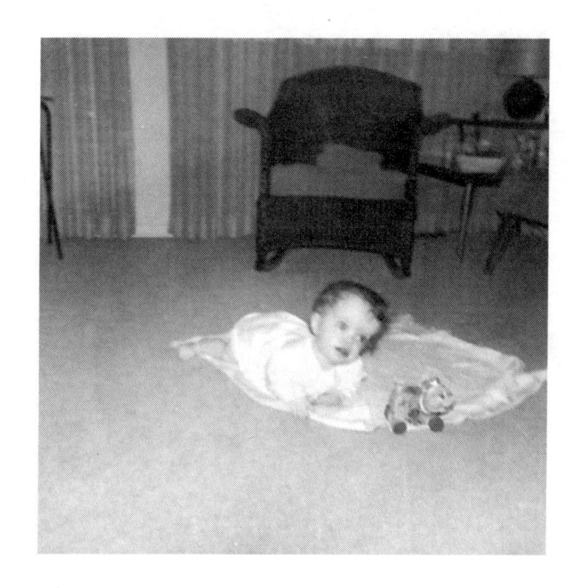

One of the earliest pictures of me.

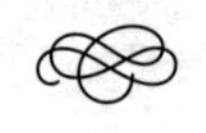

Chapter 2

I would stand tall and be proud of what I am

My awareness that I was any different from my siblings or friends happened gradually. By age eight or nine, I knew I was tinier than others but really didn't comprehend why people stopped, stared, or called me "midget." I recall asking my mom why I was being called "midget" and she simply explained the word meant small. At the time, that was the only explanation I seemed to need. There would be many more opportunities to ask my parents similar questions as time went by.

By this particular age, I knew where to line up when my class was required to line up from tallest to shortest. My best friend during this time was also of shorter stature, so I didn't feel isolated or singled out. I knew that most clothes purchased for me had to be hemmed. I was different, but I didn't feel different. I felt special.

For the majority of my elementary school years, I ignored the differences and was determined to participate in everything my peers were accomplishing. Academically, I found most assignments in school easy to complete and loved to assist others because my work was completed quickly. During recess play, I always seemed to be a part of a going group that formed private clubs with secret passwords and meetings. I also loved participating in track and field days and field trips. It was extended outdoor social time with my friends. I didn't hesitate in trying to compete in most events even though the races I participated in took twice as long while others waited for me to finish. I thought it was weird that as I finished a race, there would be more clapping for my last-place finish than for those who had won the race. My focus was ensuring I completed the event to earn points for my team.

The one field event that seemed to challenge me, however, was the high jump competition. For the safety of the participants, they brought in large nets containing foam blocks on which to land. These filled nets were as tall as I was and my analytical mind never did figure out how I could leap over a bar and land on top of the foam. This, to me, was one of the first times I felt I was at a disadvantage and excluded.

Our home was across the street from a large city park, and my friends and I would spend hours playing various games or exploring the ravine. Similar to others, I learned basic childhood skills including riding a bicycle and skating on our local outdoor rink. I loved playing baseball and badminton and seemed to be skilled at various eye-hand physical feats.

Our neighbourhood gangs were rich in creating games and

activities throughout the day. Most often after supper, friends would meet and play hide and seek using one of the corner power poles on the street as home base. Those evenings ended when the siren from the fire department blared out, informing children it was nine-thirty. We would quickly run home and look forward to the next day of play.

While growing up and competing with other children who were also growing, I knew I was not the most physically competent, but I wasn't concerned about it. It was during my last years in elementary school when I was about eleven or twelve years old that I started to become conscious of my differences and reluctant to continue to participate in common tasks that highlighted my incapability. That was also the beginning of my lifelong battle with weight issues. I quit moving. My perception of myself changed from focusing on what I thought was right to trying to meet what others might think would be right for me.

This realization or concern of being different, which my family strived hard to protect me from, came about from two significant milestones. The first was a series of medical appointments in Saskatoon. My body was changing, and I was experiencing unexplained knee and leg pains. The worst prescription ever prescribed for a person with dwarfism was provided to my parents by an orthopaedic surgeon who I recall was grossly overweight.

This was not the era of CT scans or MRIs. This was not the era emphasizing fitness and movement as a healthy lifestyle. The specialist made his recommendations based on X-ray images and conveyed his diagnosis to my parents and me. His diagnosis was arthritis in all my joints. He recommended to my parents that I should refrain from walking any distances and should discontinue any other physical activities that put pressure on my knees. He also said I needed to keep my weight down.

These recommendations changed a lot about me and changed in large part the way I interacted with my peers. I quit so many things, including walking with my friends to school and participating in various physical games and activities. It was also recommended I start carrying a small stool to rest my legs on while seated at the larger student desks. All of a sudden there were changes in my life into which I had no input.

For years, I was encouraged to be the same—the same as my siblings, and the same as my peers. In one quick moment, there were discussions and plans of changes that emphasized my differences from others. Ironically, about thirty years after this diagnosis I was looking into reasons why my joints were causing problems for me and mentioned to the specialist that I had lived with arthritis all my life. The ability to capture finer images of our bodies had changed by then and this specialist quickly ruled out arthritis as the reason for my symptoms. In fact, he said, he could not see any evidence of past symptoms of arthritis.

The second medical appointment long ago was with a genetic specialist I had been seeing over a number of years. That specialist was monitoring the rate of my growth and providing advice to my parents about taking care of someone who was a dwarf. The focus of this particular appointment was to explain to me the ramifications in terms of the genetic make-up in possible children I might have. The discussion centred on the chances of producing a child with dwarfism because of my own diagnosis. Since science class was an interest of mine, and we had already discussed genetic probability in school, I was quite comfortable with the discussion the professionals were sharing with me. The idea that there was a twenty-five per cent chance that my child would not survive birth if both parents had achondroplasia was remote for me because I had no concept, or plans, to seek a relationship with a male at that time and especially with a male who had dwarfism.

The bomb dropped when we arrived at the last item needing to be discussed during this particular appointment. This was a pronouncement that influenced me for over twenty-five years. The doctor confidently shared that the probability of me still being alive past the age of forty was minimal, as most Little People died by the time they were forty.

Today, I try to envision a young pre-teen hearing this type of information and wonder if they would have the same ability to ignore the doom and gloom of that statement. As a teenager, I was already experiencing the typical paranoid, emotional swings of adolescence and then I experienced this.

I do not recall whether my parents, particularly my mom, argued this dire prediction, but I do know that pronouncement wasn't made to be a big deal in our family. Unfortunately, it had been said, and for a large part of my life, left for me to believe. Many times when I was being encouraged to be like the norm and go out and find a special someone or even consider having children, that prediction of how long I would be part of this life scared away my dreams. Why would I place that expected grief on others? I already knew there was a high chance that my parents and siblings would have to grieve my passing earlier than others. Why would I do that to others I also loved?

My understanding of whom others thought I was started to sink in. I had heard of other Little People by this time, including opportunities to view TV personalities such as Billy Barty, an influential Little People of America (LPA)[1] personality, on television. Occasionally, when I was younger, I would be with my mother when she stopped to talk to one particular older Little Person on Main Street. She and her husband owned a small motel in our community, and to me she was a well-dressed, skinny little adult. At that time, I had little to no understanding of the various forms of dwarfism.

I knew by then that I was different and I knew I was diagnosed as having achondroplasia, but I had no real visual understanding of what Little People looked like to others. I really did not perceive myself as any different from my siblings or peers other than I stood shorter than them. I was not one who would stand for any time in front of a mirror and am still that way. I was taught swimming by a lifeguard who also was a Little Person, but again I did not have a lot of understanding about the connotations of being a dwarf. I knew I was not comfortable being near those who looked so much like me, but really did not know why.

The most significant and lasting memory that did create chaos in my perception of myself happened within this similar time period of awareness. Our church hosted a Brownie troop and I had been a member for many years. The leader I had at this time was a kind, motherly type who was always taking us on planned excursions or explorations. To this day, I believe her intent was sincere, yet she had no idea of the impact of her actions. It is a day that remains vivid to me. It was the day I was forced to meet and acknowledge other Little People.

Our Brownie troop travelled by car two blocks away from our church to the parking lot of a local supermarket. Situated in the parking lot was a long trailer temporarily placed there with ropes identifying and guiding participants where to enter and leave the trailer. There was a lineup outside and our group eagerly awaited our turn to enter the trailer. The inside of the trailer reminded me of our local museum in that it included various displays with rope barriers indicating where you could walk.

I had already figured out that this was only going to be a look-and-see tour and probably would soon be over, as the trailer really wasn't that large. Inside, we walked by a bedroom and there was a low, little bed, with a smaller dresser and end table. My first inkling that things were not right was viewing a framed picture on the wall of the bedroom. It was a picture of a family and all the members were dwarves. I really have no memory of walking through the hallway looking into other rooms until we reached the last room of the trailer.

In addition to the display of a mini-sized table, chairs and kitchen appliances there was also living room furniture in this last area. My breathing became panicky and all I wanted to do was leave. I knew what I was looking at; I just didn't want to look.

There sitting on a rocking chair was an older female Little Person completing some craft while streams of people walked by staring at her. I was heading toward the exit door when she raised her head and noticed me. It happened so fast. She came over, lifted the rope barrier, grabbed me, and guided me to a chair on the other side of the rope. I was in shock. Now I was one of them, sitting, watching as my troop and strangers stared at me.

I recall seeing a male member of that family on display joining us and speaking to me, but I have no memory of what was said. I am not really sure how long I sat there before I raced out of the trailer and hid in the car waiting for the others to return.

To this day I wonder many things: why would anyone allow himself or herself to be put on display in that manner? Was this field trip pre-planned and engineered by my Brownie troop leader for my benefit? Why would any adult supervising the safety of a group of children allow a complete stranger to manhandle and move a child into a situation where he/she no longer felt safe?

To me, this trailer exhibit was a freak show that could have been included at a state fair, which I had only read about. Throughout my years, I have been witness to similar incidents involving Little People and felt similar feelings of disgust for individuals who allow themselves, or others, to be put on display for profit.

In the late 1990s, there was a touring group of Little People males making their income by playing basketball against elementary students of various schools. The school I was teaching in was hosting one of those events and the possibility of me skipping out to avoid viewing the show didn't seem to be a choice.

Basketball is a game I know well. Back in high school, it was evident that this was a sport I would not be participating in. I became an expert on the rules and would referee the scrimmage games during gym classes. That knowledge of the game was useful years later when I volunteered to coach, along with other teachers, the girls' basketball elementary teams at one particular school.

Two things happened while watching this particular exhibition. It confirmed my belief that this was not a group of men who were skilled in the sport of basketball; instead, they were clowns. Their slapstick aerobics and juvenile antics brought great entertainment and humour to the audience. Unfortunately, their presence also changed the perspective of those present around me. I felt as if I was suddenly under examination. The students and my professional peers, who up until that time I felt had treated me without judgement, were witnessing each response I was exhibiting.

All of a sudden I felt I had become one of those men in front of us, who were not showing off their intellectual skills or professional competencies but instead providing a show for entertainment's sake. To me, they were small people, not Little People.

As a teenager, I avoided certain TV times when I knew midget wrestling was being shown. The classic 1939 movie *The Wizard of Oz* was repeatedly shown on television and I worked hard each time to avoid watching it.

In my era of childhood, the Little People celebrities I knew of were comedians. It has only been recently that the public has acknowledged the education and respected talents of Little People through media interest and social networking. The younger communities of Little People today are wiser and much more proactive in educating others of their personal rights.

History is full of stories of Little People providing entertainment for the public, and many of their journeys have been written down. One particular book, *In Our Hearts We Were Giants*, by Yehuda Koren and Eilat Negev,[2] gives the reader a unique insight to the factual story of seven dwarves of the Ovitz family who survived the Holocaust during World War II using their entertainment skills.

"Entertaining the masses" is a saying I acknowledge to myself when I am present in front of those who, to me, want me to be small. I have mastered the skill of being small and can turn on my performance skills without hesitation. As a young adult, I would show off my skills by emphasizing the physical differences that allowed me to display unique parlour tricks, such as rising up from a floor position without bending my legs, or lifting my straight leg up to my head so that my foot would reach my mouth.

Others, even today, continue to encourage me to reiterate a unique story of difference or interaction that might provide humour or entertainment for the strangers in the room. If I object to those performances, I am judged and regarded in a negative fashion. Instead, the minute I start speaking a switch is turned on, my feelings are turned off and the objective is to entertain and provide a positive experience for the listener. That is not me, but that is a me I can be.

I am pleased that societal change has taken place and current public "LP" personalities are sharing their intellect and values that better represent the majority of Little People. However, a battle for respectful acknowledgement and physical accommodations continues. Little People continue to advertise false talents or skills that have nothing to do with bringing dignity or respect to our culture. Horrific events such as dwarf tossing continue to be advertised as an entertainment/sporting event in some communities.

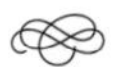

That period of adolescent change long ago, along with other experiences, influenced my perception of myself. How I perceived others viewed me at that time changed to the negative in a significant way. Combine that with the medical specialist's misdiagnosis and normal influence while entering into my middle years of schooling, and it created a shift in my world that I would spend a lifetime fighting against. I am really amazed that I made it through that particular segment of life in the manner I did.

Attending middle school and entering the teenage years is challenging for most, but add additional challenges or limitations and it becomes horrendous. Moving from my secure elementary school where everyone knew me to the larger junior high school with strangers increased my awareness and sensitivity to others gawking and judging my differences.

As an adult, having taught that particular age of student, I know now that every adolescent making those changes into adulthood experiences similar emotions and drama. An adolescent's intensity and degree changes depending upon the individual's circumstances. I also understand as an adult how cruel and intentional middle-school children can be in judging and excluding others who are different.

I remember the day I quit riding my bike. I loved riding my bike; the independence and speed of moving made me part of the group. But riding a bike with fixed side wheels (training wheels) for balance was no longer cool. I remember the day I quit skating—again, something I had enjoyed participating in because of the movement, the rhythm and speed. My doctor's choice for me to quit that particular activity was not mine. Our choices or opportunities in life define us. I didn't quit everything I was doing, but I feel I did quit believing I was the same as everyone around me.

In the school system all those years ago, counselling and emotional supports were available but I did not ever seek help. My parents, at one point, encouraged me to attend Provincial Little People functions organized in order for dwarf children to meet our physical peers. But I had no interest and was greatly agitated if any mention of attending events was made. Instead, I just moved forward and ignored hidden anger and negative emotions that would eventually make themselves known during other non-related challenges of life.

Perception of height is just that, a perception. I do not think about how short I am or how different I am unless actual physical limitations, unexpected incidents, or rude people present it to me. I know that those truly close to me do not judge or recognize my differences.

Today, one of my favourite moments is when my family or friends are ignoring me and they don't notice simple times when I need vertical assistance, such as when we are walking along a high buffet table filled with food. They usually apologize and intervene as needed, but their ignorance of my need or difference has always been a compliment for me. My eyes view people who are primarily of average height and I tend to judge others by their internal motivations, particularly by their actions and the demeanour they exhibit. I feel the most comfortable when those viewing me are not seeing those physical differences.

Being proud of who you are means that you need to first acknowledge the differences that make you unique and choose whether those differences are going to define you or defeat you. Being proud of who you are means, at times, to accept the limitations you are given and to quit fighting to be what you think others believe you are. Physically, I became aware that I was never going to stand vertically tall and needed to find different ways I could stand tall in front of others.

It was not an overnight solution. Instead, it has been a lifetime of solutions. An understanding I came to long ago and continue to believe in is to look outward and to concentrate on those around me. That defines who I am. I stand tall when I am doing for others. I stand tall when others are doing for me. My standing tall has nothing to do with who I am physically. My standing tall has nothing to do with experiences of my past. My standing tall is dependent upon how I am feeling about my current situations, my current relationships and my physical well-being.

I can stand tall and am proud of who I am

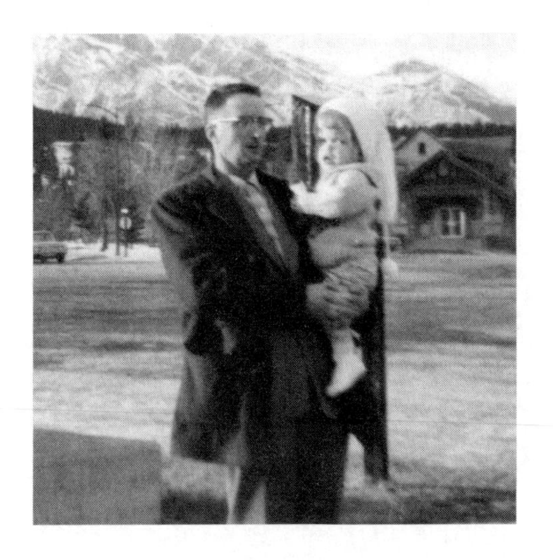

Dad and me, taken in British Columbia.

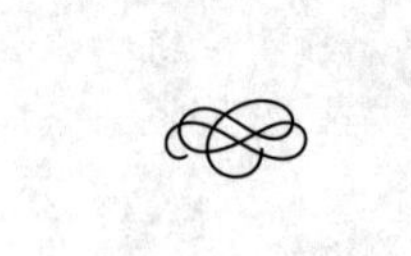

Chapter 3

Instead my life is wasted and I look back in pain

When I was growing up, I loved to watch any medical show and I continue today to enjoy a variety of TV series with reoccurring themes and constant characters. As a child, watching *Marcus Welby, M.D.,*[3] *Emergency!*[4] and *M*A*S*H*[5] were my lifelines, my hope. I would watch them faithfully, thinking that someday they would show a medical miracle to help change me.

It was only as an adult that I realized I was really searching for more than one type of change. Of course, I was seeking change in my body image, but also change in my relationships with others, change in my abilities and change in my loneliness. My interest in these shows may also have been the possibility of a chosen interest in a medical profession as an adult. The fact that I pass out when seeing bodily fluids definitely steered that path to alternate career plans.

Growing up, I wished at times that I were different for other reasons. If I was going to be noticed I wanted to be noticed for qualities other than my stature. However, the reality of the stares, the name-calling and the attention during certain periods of my life overwhelmed me and I needed a time-out. So I used the fantasy of TV stories and movies to draw me away from my realities and continued in an instilled belief that someday there would be a miracle medical cure for me.

Watching the buildup of drama, with the expectation that within an hour a miracle would occur, was very addictive. Being engaged in activities such as TV watching or today's equivalent, playing digital online games, did nothing to create solutions to life problems, but it did provide an escape from reality.

Living in my parents' home, I was not given the choice of hiding and blanketing myself away from others for very long. I look back and realize my parents did allow times when I needed to vegetate, but soon I was required to get up and complete tasks similar to what my siblings were accomplishing. I have always wondered if all parents of Little People growing up were like mine, determined and adamant that my life would mirror the norm of others. I do not know, but I believe I was one of the fortunate ones.

My favourite line is from a film I own titled *Unconditional Love.*[6] This movie is about a housewife's obsession for a particular famous singer and her journey to discover herself while she discovers who the singer is after he is murdered in the city she lives in. In one particular scene, the actor Kathy Bates (the housewife) is admonishing the character portrayed by Rupert

Everett (the singer's partner) who is sharing his impressions about how society views him for being gay. She is telling him that his worries are insignificant as compared to her daughter-in-law's situation, who in the storyline is a dwarf.

Whenever I need a feeling-good fix, I watch this movie. It could be classified as a musical or a comedy, two of my favourite genres. In addition to the witty and intelligent storylines, this was the first movie that portrayed the role of a dwarf, especially a female, as competent, honest and aggressive to those that treated her unfairly. The actor Meredith Eaton's line, "They never stop noticing me," startled me as I watched this video for the first time. That was so, so true. Her curt response to someone staring at her in public, "Why don't you take a picture? It will last longer!" has been a silent mantra I have voiced in my head for years but have never expressed orally, as it would not be socially appropriate.

In addition to having to explore and accept who I was during my developing years, I was also faced with the challenge of justifying to others that I really was Linda Nelson, daughter of Ellie and Richard Nelson. As I said earlier, for others to mistake me for someone else was very common and continues to happen to this day.

One of my first memories of this misidentification happened when I was in my fourth year of elementary school. In school, I at times volunteered to help teachers during recesses so I could avoid the running and playing activities on the playground. Sometimes I was tired of the attention and differences from others. Sometimes I was just tired of trying to keep up with my peers. I also think my interest in teaching and working in schools later in life came about because of this opportunity for a real break.

Back then, if there weren't any teacher preparation tasks available I would persuade my mom to write a note so I could stay at my desk and draw. I suspect now that my need for escape was probably also due to discomfort of undiagnosed spinal problems that were not addressed until I reached my forties. I now know that those periods of stillness and quiet were probably a time to heal for me, but at nine years of age I simply knew I didn't have the energy to go out and play.

It was during one of those times that the first of a series of related incidents occurred. I was sitting at my desk in the front row in the grade three classroom. It was recess time, and I was the only one in the room. I noticed a group of young men lean into the room, look at me and then continue walking down the hall. I can't recall the exact number of men, but there were certainly three, maybe more.

A few minutes later, these strangers returned to my classroom, knelt down in a half circle around my desk, and greeted me by a name that wasn't mine. This was an age when I had started noticing that others sometimes addressed me in my hometown by another name. I stated I wasn't "Helen" (a fictitious name). One of them then said to me, "You are our sister, Helen."

I started to panic and said louder that I wasn't Helen. They argued with me and the volume of their words got louder. The tallest one, I assume he was the oldest, leaned towards me and reached for me saying, "Come on, Helen, it's time to go."

I don't think he ever touched me because by then, I had started screaming at them. I don't recall the exact words I said but the observations shared by staff members who had heard the commotion said I had told them to "Get the hell out of my classroom."

As a young child you sustain emotions and for me the emotion I recall is fear: fear of a group of young men who were tall and thin with dark hair; fear of walking to school alone; fear of sitting in a classroom by myself; fear of old postal delivery vans.

My family spent a lot of time talking about the incident, and while I believe they thought I was beyond hearing range, one of the things I heard was that one of the brothers from this incident drove a parcel delivery van. By coincidence or my paranoia, I started noticing a red and white postal van idling at the corner across the street numerous times.

This was when I started finding reasons to be driven to school even though we only lived one block away. My fears eventually abated, and while I kept a vigilant watch for tall, thin men with dark hair, I soon returned to my normal routines of playing and interacting with others on the playground. But my trust in approaching strangers was forever altered.

The second incident happened a few years afterwards. I used to love attending our local Fair Days held during the summer. My favourite activities were riding the Ferris wheel and the roller coaster, as well as jumping inside the large balloon tent. On that particular day, I was with a friend, and we had just exited the jumping tent. A young man approached me, at first I was not afraid. He seemed younger than his brothers who had previously approached me, and his hair was a lighter colour. He called me by that same name from years ago, and told me I was going with him. Once more, I have little recollection of my reaction other than recalling my mom taking me home soon afterwards from the fair.

It didn't end. For a few years after that, a particular young girl would approach me periodically outside of my junior high school and tell me how I was adopted and had been taken from her family. By this time, my knowledge of who had given birth to me and whom I belonged to was firm. I tended to ignore her or others in the community who continued to address me with this name of "Helen." Inside, however, there was still the occasional doubt, with the question "what if they are right?" Especially during moments when I was in emotional battles with myself, this experience did not help in my quest to figure out who I was.

My feelings from that time for the real Helen were full of heartache and sympathy. How awful would it be to not only be as different as an LP, but also have the additional challenge of an unstable home life? Her brothers were dealing with their own hurt of having a sister removed from their home and their actions reflected the only way they knew how to solve their problem. I was so fortunate to be part of a family that, while we are not totally in agreement with each other, definitely will protect and support each other in need.

The conclusion of this story was provided to me a while back. I was attending an LP conference in another province and somehow found out that the real "Helen" was present at the hotel hosting the conference. I secretly scouted her out. A friend of mine, who knew her, helped me identify her amongst the crowd of other Little People in the hotel foyer. I was expecting many similarities in stature, facial features, etc. If her brothers could easily misidentify myself as their sister when we were children, would it not make sense that we would be physically similar as adults? Far from it; maybe as children there might have been some similar body features, but thirty-five years later there were huge discrepancies including our height, body size and stature.

I did not approach her and identify who I was, or share with her those experiences of long ago. I felt that identifying myself to this person would have had no purpose. She was not the cause of my fear or my anxieties from these childhood incidents. Just by being there in front of me she reaffirmed that the incidents did occur and that I hadn't imagined them. She also, without her awareness, assisted in getting me past the fears that were induced from the childhood experience.

The mislabelling of my name and the insistence that I am somebody I am not is continuous, yet separated through time. The repetition of this occurrence increases the farther away I am from my home community. Being called a different name has even happened in my home. I have answered my door to strangers and once viewed, have been engaged again in the recurring conversation of persuasion, trying to prove I am not the person the inquirer thought I was.

I have always wondered, is this normal? I have once in a while mistakenly called out to a stranger who is walking by me assuming he or she is someone I know. But I have never challenged that stranger, asking numerous personal questions for identity purposes. Instead, I quickly notice the physical differences after a second look and apologize for my error.

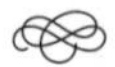

During our adolescence, we tend to be self-centred on the continual changes that are happening to us physically, socially and emotionally. Physically, for me, the discrepancy of height was growing ever more distinct, and I became more cognizant of those differences between my friends and myself. I continued to be accepted by my peers, but the rules of that acceptance seemed to change. I did not seem to share the same interests, and tended to regard myself as somewhat more immature than my classmates. Emotionally, my abilities to cope with my physical changes seemed to be overwhelming, and I preferred focussing on my interactions with my friends, my schooling and my goals of a career, instead of addressing the pain I absorbed because of my differences.

As a teenager and young adult, I would mask the emotional disappointment of not being part of the norm and instead would portray to others a presence of determination and drive. As a student in high school, I chose safe activities and clubs to be involved in such as photography or yearbook. I preferred being the one behind the camera. My role within the drama club was always behind the scenes, ensuring that I was part of the group I wanted to be included in, but having no focus or attention on me.

The same is true for my musical abilities while growing up. Whether it would be playing the piano or singing in the church choir, I preferred being in the background where others wouldn't notice me, and preferred not to participate in any solos, recitals or examinations that would bring direct attention upon me.

As a high school student, and later as a young adult, I worked hard in creating an image of a competent, caring individual who had goals and expectations. I graduated from high school and started my journey to become a teacher.

But I never let go of my dream for a miracle. The fantasy, or now a fascination, of being taller, continues. Today, it is usually a fleeting thought that passes through my consciousness during certain life activities. Living now with medical challenges, including symptoms that exist because of my bone structure, is the exception to the sense of fleeting. Writing this book has been another exception. So currently, my awareness and fantasies are rather prevalent.

My recurring fantasy didn't involve any medical intervention. It was based on a dream. Lying in bed, I am in a full body stretch. I see my limbs lengthening, and I believe I am growing taller with each stretch. I believe I can hop up out of bed (I've never hopped before), and continue my day as an average-height person, preferably five-feet, six-inches tall. That's the height I always regarded as perfect for a woman.

A different fantasy occurs at times when I am climbing up onto a stool or a chair and turn around to face an open room. This raised perspective is so different, and I pause to think that this is what my family and friends are seeing. The upper kitchen cupboards that usually tower over me don't seem as daunting. I ponder how hard it would be to bend down and reach something from the floor. I notice items such as mirrors and wall hangings. But I am missing things as well. I no longer notice the minute dust bunnies in the corners of the room. I can no longer see into the back of a lower cabinet. And I always wonder what would happen if I just took a step forward, a step off that stool.

While moving through my teenage years into adulthood, there were many aspects of my life that were within the norm. I continued being a student who passed all her classes and was focussed on achieving a particular career. I continued my involvement in music lessons and different social organizations. I moved through different social networks of friends depending on my current interests. I worked in part-time jobs. I strived so hard to be the same as others, but life itself no longer allowed for that.

The pain of this twenty-three-year-old who wrote a poem about how her life was wasted is now so easily understood. My life growing up was different, and while I was coping with the challenges and changes that most young adults were encountering, I saw myself missing out on important milestones my family members and friends were achieving.

I was included, but felt so excluded because of the differences. Others around me were growing up and maturing into adults. I couldn't help but compare myself to others and viewed myself as lacking the skills and abilities to succeed as "normal."

The poem was written while I was in my second year of teaching. With the exception of a fellow teacher, who was single and female, I had made close friendships with many married couples within the small community where I was working. I felt accepted, included, and assumed my status was equal to the others in this social group. But that was not the case. It became clear that my lack of having a spouse or partner created a secondary status. I was the wife's companion, the husband's acquaintance, but never the couple's friend. If the couple were entertaining other couples then I, and other single people, were excluded. It didn't occur to me that this was just an antiquated tradition of this particular community. In my perception, it was a dawning realization that it was my relationship status, not my height differences, that were part of the criteria for inclusion. But I was personally blaming my height status for all my perceived grievances with my life.

While growing up, I have had many people surrounding me, providing the encouragement and positive energy to sustain my outlook of life. My need for those supports from others continues, but there were times when the emotional negative influences of situations and events changed my way of thinking. This negative thinking started a battle within that I have worked hard not to dwell on, and have preferred to ignore for a large part of my life. Looking back in pain is a dark place for me, and I choose not to enter that doom and depression unless I am unexpectedly placed there for a reason or circumstances that require those types of reflections.

Emotional darkness, for me, has been a time when I have melted down, screaming and crying and asking, "Why? Why was I born this way? Why did this happen to me? Why can't I be like others? Why do I see what is inside me as so normal, but why can others only see what is on the outside?"

I truly believed others would not notice me as much if I had been born with a different physical ailment, such as having to be in a wheelchair or lacking a sensory ability like vision or hearing. I even pondered how an older family friend who had Down's syndrome coped with being different, and often assumed that her lack of higher cognition allowed her peaceful ignorance of this pain.

A significant dark time for me were moments when I would ask myself three distinct questions, and the answer was always the same for each question. "Who are you?" "What are you?" "What will you always be?" A midget.

It's a word I hate, a word that has been said to me in hate, a word that I will continue to fight against forever. It was never said in wonderment or love. It was said to classify, to label, to help justify the fear of the person who was saying it to me or to others. It is an outdated use of a word that for me has never been said with peace or joy. Just like the long-ago use of words to describe minority races, or other words people find offensive, to say that word in any context in reference to a Little Person or within the presence of an LP in today's society is deemed highly inappropriate and will certainly be addressed.

I have presented a strong wall to others where I would pretend to brush off the use of the word. I have instructed the name-sayer that the "M word" only meant small, and maybe if they really wanted to offend me they should try calling me something else. But I *was* offended. To be called a name that doesn't allow me any control over its connotation is the most offensive. Call me "fat" and I have a choice to lose weight. Call me a "bitch" and I have a choice to be kinder to others. But when you call me the "M word" there are no choices. I cannot change that facet of my existence. I cannot hide or mask it. At my lowest of lows, that was the one word, especially self-directed, that would succeed in bringing me down.

This significant moment with the writing of the poem was a culmination of all the unexpressed stresses and anxieties I was experiencing. This was also the beginning of a self-deprecating, non-supportive action that would further dig that hole of depression. I would let myself take inventory, and would start listing all the physical malformations I had. The funny thing was that even though this action was repeated whenever the hole opened up and started to swallow me, I never did accomplish the goal of listing all my perceived disfigurements. I usually started at the top of my head and worked down, but rarely got halfway down my body before the number of malformations I perceived far outweighed my energy and current emotional stability to write them down.

Many of the features I deemed negative at that time were changeable— my weight and body image, for example. I was heaviest as I left my university days and entered into teaching. Sitting still and only studying and eating for four years did not help. I did not participate in regular exercise, and had no clue that the endorphins to help prevent depression are increased by physical movement. I stayed inside a lot and did not understand benefits from the natural sunshine's ability to alleviate sadness. I did not eat right and had no awareness of how certain sugars and fats influence one's negative emotions.

Common to others with achondroplasia, my front teeth protruded because of the inequality of space in my mouth as compared to the number of teeth. The choice to have my teeth straightened as a teenager was briefly considered by my parents but not carried out after being told that the shape of my mouth wouldn't retain the shape of highly expensive straightened teeth. Years later, in my thirties, I ignored that continued advice and chose to change the look of my smile. The simple action of removing four teeth provided the necessary space to reduce the extreme overbite.

I was alone teaching for the first time in a community that had never been subject to having someone as different as I was. For the first time in my life, I was lacking the constant support of my family and close friends. For the first time, it wasn't my parents pressuring me, but me trying to lose weight. I had become tired of explaining myself and tired of the repetition of teaching others about dwarfism.

I was an emotional mess. I truly believed that no one else could relate to this pain; I was crushed that this, my life, had happened to me. I needed to stop this spiral of downward emotion and started to question what worked for me. I needed to step away from the darkness and refrain from always looking back.

Looking back, I realize that I was so young, lacking the insights and values that are gained with maturity and experience. My perspective at that time was centred on me. But I also knew that this was not me. I did not want to live in a negative world of blame and self-deprecation. I expected and wanted a better life.

Pain, whether it is emotional or physical, is an indicator of a need for change. To step away from the darkness and refrain from always looking back, I need to continue to change and create different goals.

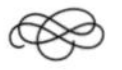

Setting goals and deadlines gives a person purpose. Setting goals moves your forward, letting go of what is holding you back. I love goals. Daily I write out plans and "to do" lists. I even like sharing them with others. It sustains my need for direction, focus and purpose. It organizes my day and ensures that my promises to others are not missed. At my current age, it also allows me to refer to them when I sometimes forget what I am supposed to be doing.

For me to climb out of that abyss long ago and for future times of emotional challenges, I became a connoisseur of self-help philosophies. I started studying particular authors and attending professional development sessions that focussed on teaching me how to find solutions. My professional duties in Special Education and Gifted Education during my early teaching years gave me reasons for this expansion of knowledge. I became trained in various personality types, creative problem solving, multiple levels of solution focused therapy and cognitive coaching. It was easy to justify to others the need to gain additional knowledge for the sake of my career. But looking back at my acquisition of training and knowledge during those years, a large majority of my learning was for my personal well-being.

Everything I did to this point to help relieve the emotional pain was done in private. As I coped in my adult years with the varying challenges of differences, I found, however, that my perspective of how I was viewing my circumstances was sometimes off kilter. I would never admit to myself, or even identify to others, that my perceptions were out of alignment. It was usually the degree of negative aggression I expressed or put upon others that would trigger my awareness that maybe other supports such as a qualified counsellor were needed.

Eventually, I had to acknowledge that there were times during some challenges in my life that reaching solutions needed to include outside supports. The majority of these supports were usually sought out during a significant milestone such as the passing of a loved one or when a personal medical issue was overwhelming. The stigma, even as a teacher, in receiving emotional support by a trained counsellor could be detrimental in how others regarded you professionally. Eventually, though, I acknowledged my need for support and ignored the possible implications or consequences of having others know of this need. I was fortunate during my career to have the emotional health support of the Saskatchewan Teachers' Federation (STF).[7] Counsellors travelled to our communities and met with teachers in very private settings.

The hardest step of any change is the first one. Making a phone call requesting counselling support is daunting and very frightening. It is not the possibility that others would know what you need, it is the fear in admitting that you are unable to solve this certain challenge on your own.

I have usually walked into these planned therapy sessions with an agenda of control. Me, the one with the problem, would be deciding what topics were going to be discussed and what issues I was needing to address. If the counsellor was a proficient one, they would usually allow me the time to lead the first few sessions nattering on about issues that were not the issue. Eventually, the professional in the room would do the work they were trained in and guide me to what I really should be focussing on.

Counselling for me has been a tool that would bring me back to seeing more than one perspective: back to seeing beyond my needs, back to others seeing the me I want to be. Everyone copes with challenges in life – that is part of being human. It is how we approach and deal with those challenges that determines who we are and who we have the potential of becoming.

Those who have experienced trauma or grief typically follow an emotional path including disbelief, guilt, anger, depression and eventual acceptance. Most, in time, work through the stages and move on from their traumatic experience in some way. I am starting to believe that I have probably experienced recurring trauma throughout my life and have failed to recognize those experiences as trauma. As well, I have ignored the needed stages of healing.

Pain itself is a perspective. My perception of pain has changed. I still cope with pain, but it has become more of a priority to address the physical challenges than the emotional ones. The preventative health requirements to keep me from having further major surgeries are an important part of my day. My quest to live independently and move independently is a priority. The need to interact with others and give of myself to others is a life's journey.

My life is full and I can look back with pride, celebration, interest, and joy

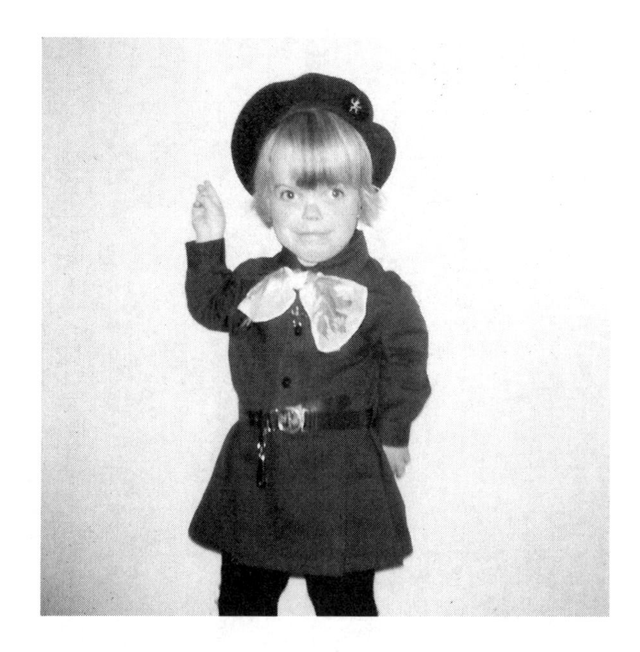

Dressed in my Brownie uniform.

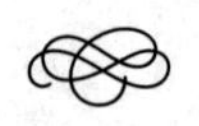

Chapter 4

The pain of my family, the selfishness and greed

Growing up, my family was a constant for me. For the first ten years or so, the nine of us fit into an ordered household sharing chores and responsibilities. My parents were the conductors of this ensemble with my siblings each taking a part to create harmony and unique melodies of their own.

The two oldest siblings were the ones to provide additional emotional and physical parental support for my younger sister and me. They were our secondary caregivers and spent a lot of time raising us. My memory of the spankings I received as a child sees my sister being the primary one giving that discipline. When I needed help with a challenge, whether it be a physical one or someone to wipe my tears, I saw my brother always there to rescue me. The roles those two elders took on so long ago in their teenage years continued throughout our lifetime.

My oldest sister, Allison, the nurse, never let go of the fact that I was different. She was the one in the family who asked the pointed questions about celebrities who were Little People. Ally would invite me, in front of her friends, to tell the unique stories of my life for entertainment purposes. She let me talk incessantly about incidents of being short. Ally surrounded me with the medical care and personal interest in me being a dwarf that I seemed to be seeking whenever we had an opportunity to visit.

My oldest brother, Michael, who currently lives on the farm homestead, lived in the basement of our home in town longer than any of us as we were growing up. My best times with Mike were sitting inside the massive combine or perched on a wheel well within a tractor cab chattering throughout the day. Mike was my sounding board, and I would seek him out when I needed someone to help me look at life from a different perspective.

The middle brother and sister, to me, were the rebels of the family throughout their teenage and young adult years. They seemed to be perpetually changing and challenging the order of our family. Both were very smart and outgoing and their daredevil antics as teenagers made for memorable storytelling for years afterwards. These two siblings influenced me to be like them – independent, creative and assertive.

My middle brother, Lyle, the jack-of-all-trades, held similar beliefs to my mother's of creating normalcy in our family and displayed minimal attention to my particular needs. My memories of Lyle as a child are of his time on the farm, and the hours he put in working on old vehicles in front of the garage. I was fascinated with how Lyle could fix anything, and if he didn't know how, he would work to find the answers. For many years, I found myself often seeking Lyle's time and acceptance but for the most part feeling regarded as a lesser priority. Today, he continues his interest in sharing his time with others and supporting many family members, particularly the next generations. We have struggled at times as siblings to communicate but are able to be present together when others are in need.

My early memories of my middle sister, Nicole, the office manager, is that she spoke with lots of volume, moved quickly when walking and drove with speed. I watched Nic from afar as she grew into an adult and wanted to be so much like her. I especially loved listening to Nicole practice the piano. When I had moved away to enter university, my mother decided during that first year of schooling to convert my upstairs bedroom into a TV/sewing room. During my second summer home, Nic offered me a bedroom in the house she was renting on the other side of the city. I recall that Nic's outgoing personality and efficiency with whatever she was doing was addictive for me, and I would follow whatever plans or ideas she wanted.

My mother devoted many of her years to the battles that needed to take place to ensure my independence and my well-being as a child growing up. Nicole took over this role when I encountered health issues in my forties and needed to win the biggest battle of all with our provincial government. My challenge with this sister is keeping the balance in terms of doing for each other and making sure I am doing my share.

The youngest boy in our family, Gregory the architect, was older than me and while he was not regarded as one of the younger kids, he was also not seen as a middle child. Greg's unique status was reflective of who he became as an adult. As a child, Greg would invite me to play baseball with his friends, and would camp outside in our back yard with me overnight in an old green, stinky tent. Greg also taught me through childhood experiences to keep up and to stand up for myself.

Greg and I have a relationship of distance now. He is busy with his family and his profession in a large city community. Unlike some other siblings that prefer keeping in contact and checking in, Greg is comfortable in the once-every-few-years chats or visits we have. There remains in me a need for closer contact with him and when those opportunities happen, I feel that special bond that years ago brought comfort to me.

My little sister, Ivory, was the quiet one in our family, the library technician. She was born three years after me, but because of my late physical developments we were treated at times like twins. We were grouped together and called "the girls." Our parents carried us around together, dressed us in similar homemade outfits, and treated us relatively the same for a large part of our childhood.

Throughout my adult life, Ivory and I have lived separate lives, but we have always been connected. We stay in each other's houses when visiting, even though we both have choices of siblings to visit. The majority of holiday travelling we have done together and find that our interests complement each other. Ivory has consistently been very giving of her time to others and did not hesitate to give up an entire years' worth of holidays when I needed someone to accompany me and provide personal care after a major surgery.

My memories of our family times were moments of celebrations and gatherings. Our family was always active, always on the move and forever chaotic. My parents had a healthy balance of life and while they devoted considerable time to the farm and their children's activities, they also made time for their own interests outside of our home.

There was an expectation from our parents that we would all have some sort of proficiency in playing a musical instrument, and our parents were forever trotting us back and forth to music lessons and band rehearsals. Most of us were also involved in community group activities such as 4-H, church choirs, sport clubs, Brownies and/or Boy Scouts. We were busy, but we didn't see our life as overwhelming.

Even our meals were in some ways on a schedule. Breakfast time was usually a free-for-all with siblings scrambling to make toast or eat bowls of cereal. Dad was generally in charge of breakfasts and would treat us with special meals of pancakes, boiled eggs or my favourite, hot bread and milk. Lunches depended on who was home. Our elementary school was only a block away, and the younger ones would have plenty of time to walk home and eat lunch. Most days, during the winter times, Dad would be home and provided us with a simple hot meal such as canned soup or a baked potato. My favourite noon meal was when Mom would bake macaroni and cheese, which seemed to fall mostly on Wednesdays.

Suppers depended on which season we were in. The summers were filled with barbecue meals, most often served at the lake cabin where some of us migrated with Mom; Dad and older siblings would occasionally visit. Saturday night was traditionally waffles night until the teenage members eventually took over the kitchen area and changed it to pizza night.

During seeding and harvest times, female family members created full hearty meals that were individually packed into quart-sized casserole dishes and then wrapped in newspaper. Desserts were always prepared ahead of time. Each night, my mom or an older sibling would travel out to the farm with the boxes of packed meals to feed those who were working. The kids (typically Ivory and myself) were dragged along because we were too young to stay at home alone. I loved those times. Ivory and I either ate ahead of time at home, or we had our own pint-sized dish of food to eat on our laps while sitting on a blanket in the middle of whatever field my dad and brothers happened to be working. The smell of warmed newspapers is a unique memory that many of the siblings still recall.

Sunday our schedules came to a halt. Dad faithfully attended church, usually choosing to attend the earlier communion service. Mom and some of us would attend the later morning service where Mom would sing in the senior choir and my siblings and I would join others in the junior or intermediate choir. The noon meal generally included some form of biscuit that Mom or Dad made from scratch. Sunday evening we would all gather and celebrate with our family sitting around the extended dining room table, most often eating the traditional roast chicken meal that Mom and others had spent the day preparing.

I loved those Sunday dinners. In addition to the sense of being together with everyone present, that was the one meal when the food was brought to the table. For the majority of meals, we would sit at the kitchen table, and the younger ones were given plates of food already portioned out while my older siblings helped themselves to their food straight from the pots on the stove. For me, the privilege of dishing my own food from the stove was a rite of passage that I so much wanted but didn't actually achieve until I believe I was much older, closer to being an adult.

Our Sunday evenings commonly ended with family members joining in a game of cards such as cribbage, a sing-along around the piano with Dad playing his mandolin or just continuing our hearty conversation around the table.

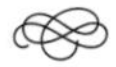

Time spent at the farm was important to me during my childhood years. The short journeys along the highway and gravel roads to reach the farm were always filled with anticipation. At times, our excitement to reach the farm was a little loud, and Mom would threaten one or all of us with the promise of stopping the car and making us walk. It was usually the morose, pouty teenagers who would sometimes challenge her a second time and they would be walking into the farmyard long after we had arrived by car.

If Dad were the driver, he would pack us in his truck and often take us along the back route approaching the farm from a different direction. We loved it and would scream loudly knowing that as he reached the top of a hill he would turn off the truck's engine. We would then coast in silence down the gravel road towards our yard.

For the younger children, the farm was our gigantic play land where we could roam and explore without scheduled time limits or restrictions. Past the curving road surrounded by trees, the yard space expanded into a circle of buildings that to me spanned several city blocks. A row of huge fuel tanks and red granaries lined the west border. The working sheds where my dad and brothers spent hours fixing and preparing farm equipment lined the east boundary. To the south were a few ancient relics of buildings, old vehicles and a gnarly windbreak that encouraged grand stories of play.

On the north side stood the original farmhouse built in the early years of the last century, the focal point of the farmyard. It was a towering two-storey building with multiple entrances into different rooms on the first floor. It had been years since anyone had lived in this house, but it was still standing and was, to me, our second home. The house was full of old furniture and relics left by previous generations. The majority of rooms were no longer in use, but when Dad's siblings and their families came to visit the entire house came alive with their stories of remembrance and the opportunities we had to stay overnight in the cold, drafty bedrooms upstairs.

Day trips to the farm were common from spring until fall with scheduled jobs planned for most of us each day. While the older siblings were driving tractors and combines or hauling grain, the younger ones were given housework duties or required to join Mom, who always seemed to be tending the garden. It didn't take long for our attention to our assigned duty to wane and we would quietly wander off to explore and play.

Traditionally, Nicole, Ivory and I became part of the bi-annual cleaning of the kitchen. While the rest of the house sat still and was rarely used, the front porch and kitchen area was my father's office and the farm workers' gathering place for coffee breaks and lunches. Once every spring and fall, Dad would transport us to the farm with the expectation that we would clean the kitchen. I always wondered why Mom never volunteered to do this role or even offer to help us. I now know why.

Those who were working the land entered the kitchen of the house in farming mode. They walked in covered with layers of dirt and mud, sat on the chairs around the table and left soon afterwards to finish whatever job they had, hopefully before the sun went down. Their focus was on the land and not on the layers of dirt or mud accumulating on the floor or the layers of grease surrounding the burners on the stove they used to prepare their meals.

There were actually two stoves in this very large open kitchen. One was a somewhat modern electric stove and the other was an old-fashioned wood-burning stove that had a reservoir to heat up water. After Dad carried in buckets of water from the rain barrel outside, he would light a fire in the stove and leave us girls to clean the kitchen.

This was a chore we cherished for being part of the farm, yet were reluctant to tackle, because the work involved a full day. The repeated scraping and sweeping up of the mud and dirt was always the first job. Then our roles would divide, and one of us would attack the hard-encrusted grease and dirt from flat surfaces in the kitchen while the others washed the floor repeatedly, attempting to find the original colour. Once again, there was no difference in my dad's expectation of having his daughters clean the farmhouse. Along with my sisters, I learned how to keep the stove hot by piling fresh kindling and wood into it while standing on a chair. My arm length being somewhat shorter, I had to be careful not to let the flames singe my face as I leaned in to reach. Scooping a large bucket of hot water and carefully getting down from the chair while keeping the bucket steady was completed without thought.

Our reward for cleaning the house, and at other times for accompanying Dad to the farm, was a trip to the Polar Bar for milkshakes before heading home. The Polar Bar was a corner store located in the middle of our city. It seemed to have the best ice cream. We all ordered milkshakes and would drink them for the rest of the ride home. With anything sweet, especially ice cream, Dad would quickly consume his treat and then ask the others if anyone wanted to trade. Ivory and I, being the youngest and the most gullible, would quickly take that deal, reaching out to trade an almost full milkshake for one that usually only had the dregs left. It was surprising how many times we would be caught in this trap before learning to keep our own treat for ourselves.

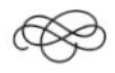

The year of my thirteenth birthday I experienced my first time of mourning the passing of a loved one. My maternal grandmother passed away from a heart attack in her own community on the West Coast. The story of her walking down a steep hill near her home to go shopping and the struggle that occurred when she attempted to return to her home reverberated within me for many years afterwards. My mother was the only one in our family who attended the funeral, and for me, things started to change in our family when Mom returned from that difficult trip.

On both sides of the family we enjoyed various relatives who had lots of character. Both of Mom's parents came from families that were part of the original 1880s settlement in the community I am now living in. Their family surnames remain familiar to many and continue to be appreciated for contributing to the development of this town, including donating the land where the local cemetery is located.

One family member I knew of was a great-aunt who lived in Alberta, Auntie G. I knew her as the "spinster" and she was regarded as somewhat of a zany individual. I understood she was my late grandfather's sister, but I never had the opportunity of meeting her in person.

Within the same year that my family had lost the only grandparent I truly got to know, many of Mom's siblings had come to our home to visit. All were quite distracted by an official document they were examining. It was a will detailing the wishes of Auntie G, who had passed within months of Grandmother's passing. With the exception of relatively small monetary gifts for my siblings, she had left her entire estate to me. Her unique wording of this gift was difficult for everyone involved to comprehend and would take some years to resolve.

Auntie G, who only knew about me, indicated that the profits from her entire estate would be made available for my education as long as I needed those funds. Upon completion of my studies, the remainder would be gifted to a named church within the city where she had resided. Once again, a lot of attention was being focussed on me. While it wasn't until a few years later that the specifics of the will would be fully explained to me, I sensed that the meetings and discussions behind closed doors were about me.

The church that was to receive the remainder of the bequeathed funds chose to challenge the wording of the will in court. I remember at that time Mom frantically trying to find my birth certificate and me having my picture taken without anyone explaining why. As a pre-teen, emotionally in conflict for many reasons including recently losing my grandmother, I once again was wrapped up in something over which I had no choice or control.

After many years, the court decided to disregard the original wishes of Auntie G and to divide all properties and value exactly in half. Many who heard about this battle were astounded that a church would take on this challenge and want more than what would be remaining after my education was completed. From the church's perspective, the wording of "as long as Linda is needing the funds for her education" was seen as vague, and potentially I could have easily chosen to extend my studies until all the funds had been used.

At sixteen years of age, after Auntie G's estate was resolved and everyone had agreed to the judgement, my parents officially told me of this inheritance. The money was put into a trust until I reached the age of eighteen. At the time, I really didn't think much of this gift of money, but looking back I wished that someone had provided me some instruction in financial planning for those two years before I had any control of the money. My father's preference and suggestion was for me to invest for the long term and not use the funds. My mother had a different view.

I think back now and wonder what value that inheritance would be today if I had followed Dad's wishes and left the original amount to gain interest. Only after four years in university, during which I freely purchased items of want and then later, as a young professional, crazily investing some of the funds into high-risk projects, did I realize I needed to seek counsel about my choices in spending.

I look back at this generous gift I was given and realize the harm of receiving something that for others would have been regarded as a salvation. My attitude towards spending and earning my own money changed. I did work summer jobs between my years of university, but only if I wanted to. I never had a need or desire to earn money while studying, which in turn isolated me socially. I became impulsive in my spending and this lack of reflection and attention at times extended into other life choices.

Our family dynamics by then were changing and I felt like I was watching a favourite sitcom disintegrate. I was so comfortable with what was, but was experiencing so many changes within my family and with me. When so many years ago I wrote the line in my poem referring to the selfishness and greed of my family, our family was in the middle of conflict. A conflict that was similar to a previous incident from the past.

The regrettable events that led to my paternal grandmother's family long ago losing a greater part of the land they had been successfully farming has been passed down through the generations. From my perspective this was an issue of trust.

On my dad's side, my grandfather was from Sweden who had migrated with his family to the state of Minnesota. He eventually alone moved north and bought land that remains a part of our family. My grandmother was a Barr Colonist[8] who with her family and others from England travelled in 1903 to Canada to seek a better life.

In addition to my great grandparents who travelled as Barr Colonists, there were also their five children: four boys and one girl, my grandmother. During World War I, three of the sons volunteered to travel and battle oppression across the seas. The youngest brother and Grandmother remained back to help with the farming. Unfortunately, one of the three brothers did not make it back. The other two brothers, who did return, came back having experienced trauma and hardship while in battle. Upon returning, they questioned the current state of the economy of farming and hired lawyers to sue the family for the loss of expected income.

Typical to any battle that is needing to be resolved by outside mediators, the winners were the lawyers and the court system, whose fees consumed most of the family's assets. The decision required the family to sell a large part of the land they had accumulated. Eventually, the two brothers who had returned moved with their own families to settle in different communities.

Our family's telling of this story always gave the hero status to those who had remained and farmed the land, while the brothers who had travelled abroad were portrayed as the villains. But I always wondered what conversations took place so long ago that created this rift. What efforts could have been made to resolve this conflict without the damage that took place?

By the time my generation existed there was only one member of this original family from the dispute left to tell the real story. He never spoke of what actually happened. This was my father's uncle, Uncle A., who lived a quiet life of farming for close to one hundred years. The youngest son, who had lied about his age to acquire his own land when the family landed in Canada, had stayed behind to farm while the brothers fought for their country. He remained on his land for the majority of his years, never marrying or having children of his own.

Uncle A. lived in an aged, shanty-type home on his original homestead, spending most evenings creating unique tools or gadgets or travelling to the city to socialize with his friends. His house did have electricity, but little else. Indoor plumbing and a furnace would never have been considered. Uncle A. used a large stove that he would fill with wood or coal to cook his meals and keep him warm at night. My tendency to sometimes live in clutter is proudly influenced by this great-uncle. His home was filled with machine parts and old items that he cherished. His kitchen table was covered with various tools, jars of food items and correspondence. There was a tiny space left for his plate and a cup.

I began to know Uncle A. when he had already reached his mid-seventies. He was a stout Englishman with a light sweater commonly worn between his dress shirt and suit coat. He wore round-wired framed glasses that usually obscured his sparkling eyes until Mom would steal his glasses and clean them for him.

The entire community seemed to know of this uncle. When he needed to purchase items or to visit his buddies his unique mode of transportation brought about much attention. After having his driver's licence taken away some years before, Uncle A. started driving his tractor to town to complete his needed tasks. Many remember the times he would tootle past as onlookers stared at this elderly gentleman steering his vintage tractor down the streets.

Most times after visiting the city shops, Uncle A. would park his tractor in front of our house to visit. He would bring Mom unique creations, and she couldn't help but wonder about their potential use. Pot holders made of old tire rubber or ladles made from used sardine cans would appear for a while in our kitchen and then magically would be lost within a short time with Mom expressing no idea what happened to these gifts when questioned. Uncle A. was well appreciated in different ways—he was most especially noted for the toffee candy he would make and give to others on an annual basis.

Years later, Uncle A. would annually move to an apartment in the city to stay in during the cold winter months. In the last few years of his life, Uncle A. was required to live in a care home. His passing, months before reaching his 100th birthday, was for me like losing a best friend. I missed him for many years afterwards.

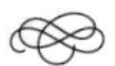

Our Sunday family dinners began changing. In my teens, I started noticing different tensions amongst the siblings and had no idea how to help heal the rifts. There was a particularly huge rift between Lyle and Nicole, who were by then young adults.

The friction whenever the two of them were present in the room was noticeable and somewhat uncomfortable for others.

I always wanted to have family meetings. When I first noticed that certain sibling relationships were not connected, I felt it would be a great idea if all of us sat at our parents' dining room table and hashed things out. It worked on television. Family members would sit down and talk out their issues with each challenge ending with a hug for each other. Our family never really talked at that level until later in life and definitely did not hug.

During a series of meals at the time of writing this particular line of this poem, a repeating theme at the table discussions was focussed on who would be taking over the family business of farming. To me, it was a given that Mike, who had farmed with Dad for close to twenty years, would slip right into that role. But other members of the family were making their intention known to be included in the business that now for the first time was showing signs of prosperity.

After one such discussion, I returned to the southern town where I was currently teaching, full of anger and distress. The heartless disregard of announcing those intentions in front of my parents, who were still contributing to the farm, and to Mike, whose life was dedicated to the farm, angered me. I regarded those who voiced this intent as selfish and greedy in their need for some control of the family business. It was as if they were already planning for the demise of our parents and arguing who was going to profit from their death.

My inability at that time to view situations from different perspectives prevented me from asking those siblings why:

"Why was it important for you to want to start being part of the farming business?" There is a love of the land and being in wide, open spaces in all my siblings. Today, I can see how missing out on being part of the land may have prompted these unexpected announcements.

My parents did not agree to their proposals and instead made the necessary financial decisions that would ensure that each of us received an equal share of their estate. They say that money is the root of evil, and while I am not one to have lived without financial means, I believe that the obsession with money can change a person. It changed me when I, without any regard, would purchase unneeded items because I could. It changed my siblings when they started monitoring and comparing to whom our parents were providing financial support.

A thread is a very delicate string that can be easily ripped apart when it becomes unravelled. I have been a part of the unravelling and contributed to weakening those threads of relationships within my family. I can stand and impart to others that I am experienced in mediating conflicts between professionals; however, I feel I have been instrumental in creating more distance rather than healing the rifts between particular family members. For many years, I felt my role in this family was to inform others. I was communicating with everyone and unfortunately not doing an effective job of it. My intention to bring others close was actually creating more distance. My attention-seeking actions were my problem, not my family's.

My perception of what my unique presence did for our family was not fully realized until many years later after writing this poem. For the most part, our family was fairly normal in the manner in which we became adults, and we were so lucky that as siblings growing up we escaped the harsh incidents of life such as fatalities or illnesses that strike others. As an adult, I wonder though—what effect did my unique presence have on my siblings' need to have a "normal" existence? Greg and Ivory, I assume, would have felt the greatest impact since our childhood friends intermingled with each other. Each sibling, though, would have his or her own perspective of living with someone who was physically different. Each would be known as the person who has a sister who is a dwarf. If I was struggling with my identity and acceptance of being normal, one can only assume my siblings also had encounters with others that would have created attention and challenges for them.

In my efforts to continually focus on my childhood family, I chose to ignore the importance of spending time creating my own adult family. I had been living my parents' family and not mine. With the aging of my parents it was only natural that this family dissipated and new generations were emerging. While my perceptions of the past have altered in so many aspects, my perception of who my family should be was strong. I was unwilling to let go of my beliefs and accept newer understandings. My siblings had all created their own families in some manner and here I was still trying to retain the only family I had experienced. I have realized that the "pain of my family" was a grieving for what was, my reluctance to recognize that grief and move on. The "selfish and greed" was also a reflection of me, not them.

Moving on also means letting go and embracing the new. New generations of our family have emerged and with each new addition there was and continues to be celebration. My time watching my nieces and nephews grow into responsible adults has been precious and important to me. They themselves have started their own families, and it is within one member of that generation this story emphasizes the importance of celebrating family.

For the last five years of Dad's life you could see the struggles he had to keep on living. His heart was failing, and he soon became a person who didn't venture far from his home. I had gotten to know more of who Dad was years earlier when we had spent time making a video montage of family pictures. I manned the camera and Dad was the narrator. Each Wednesday evening for an entire year, we would go to his basement to sort and record the many thousands of pictures. It was a time to reflect, and also a time for me to get to know this great person who had already experienced half of his life before I was born.

Dad's actual failing of life happened within days. Family members were called home and thankfully all siblings arrived in time to say our last words to him at the hospital. Mom and Ivory, who was caring for Mom, were at home the morning of Dad's death. Mom had said her private good-byes earlier and chose not to be with the crowd of family members. My oldest niece, Yvette, along with her young child and new boyfriend, arrived the morning of my dad's death. We were all sitting in a private waiting room taking turns being with Dad. I was so thankful that my grandniece, Adriana, was present. I started playing with her to distract me from my impending loss.

Within an hour of all of us gathering we were called in for a final time. We were standing beside Dad's bed and without worrying about what anyone would think I grabbed a chair and stood on it so I could be closer to him. Some were speaking to him, some were crying and I started singing. My dad was my spiritual influence, and I thought singing the Lord's Prayer was appropriate for that time.

We left the ICU room grieving, lost and wondering what to do next. Adriana, who was so new to our family as compared to others, knew what to do. She looked up and said, "Mom, they all need a hug." Adriana was right and that one gesture of giving each of us a hug in the hallway near my dad's hospital room changed us forever.

At times, I seem to ponder too much about what was and grieve greatly when changes within my family occur. Connection with family members remains important to me, and while I can understand the natural changes that take place through distance and time, I dream of the perceived closeness that existed so long ago. That is me.

I might have lost something while trying to hold on to my original family, but I believe that my family is close and will continue to change as I change. My family is a wide bevy of people that I am related to. My family is those who I connect with and trust. My family is those who ask me for assistance when they are in need, and those who don't hesitate to offer their time when I am in need. My family is the silence I experience as I live alone and my ability to embrace that silence.

The pride of my family, their accomplishments and deeds

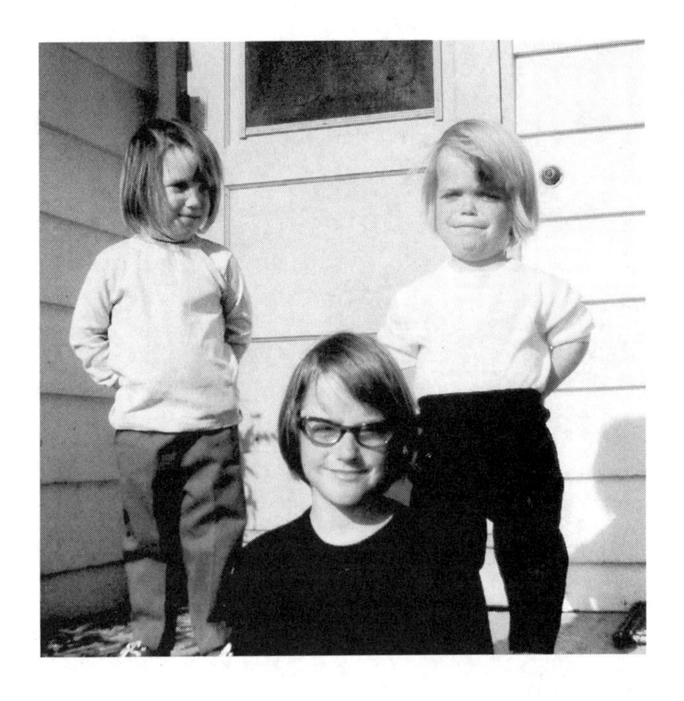

Ivory, Nicole and myself in front of our family's home.

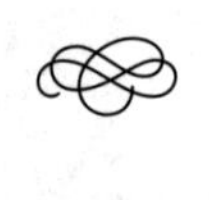

Chapter 5

The pain of my friends, the comfort and lies

My friendships have been based on my current life experiences. My childhood friends were those living near our home. They were also those at school, church or the various activities my parents involved me in. I always thought as a child that my friendships were the same as others, and I felt included. My neighbourhood friends seemed to be the most important to me as an elementary student. The closer those friends lived to me, the closer the relationships seemed to be.

One individual in particular remains a fond memory of a dear friend whose nickname was Neenie. I'm not sure at what age I first met Neenie, who was so like me, but I can guess now that we probably knew each other as infants since we were raised from birth only two houses away. She was the youngest member of her family and the second shortest person in every grade during the years that we attended school together.

Everything Neenie accomplished she did with confidence and glee. I still remember her laugh and recall she was always laughing. My memories of our time together are vague in details, but we were always playing together at school and at home. This friend was learning to tap dance and would try to teach me the steps she knew. I was so proud of Neenie, especially when I saw her dance one time on a weekly TV show that highlighted talent of young children within our province.

To me as a child, friendships were forever, and I had a hard time accepting the natural progression of change within friendship. I was eight or nine years old when Neenie's father, who was in the hotel business, moved his family to another community at the border of our province. I was miserable.

Neenie and I attempted to keep in touch for a while, but it wasn't until I was starting to attend junior high school that I realized this friendship had fallen into a different category of friendship. Upon visiting Neenie where she now lived, I was super excited to see her but common to other relationships of distance realized how much we had grown apart.

I eventually lost track of Neenie when her family once again moved to a larger city farther away. I wondered about her, though, and at times continued to reflect on this friendship of long ago, especially when watching young children dancing on a stage. Through another neighbourhood friend, Neenie and I have reconnected and in recent years exchanged occasional letters and e-mails.

As a young child and teenager, the gathering of friends was a priority, and I worked hard to make those connections. The first time I felt I was living a lie in a friendship happened when I was in my upper elementary school years. By then, I seemed to continually attach myself to kind, giving individuals. I worked hard at being included and started changing what was me inside to sustain relationships with certain friends. In the church in which I was raised, our faith was very private and rarely shared. We prayed while in church, but we rarely gathered outside the church or encouraged others to join our flock.

One particular year, a group of school friends invited me to join them at a bible school summer camp being held in a church a few blocks from our house. I knew the outside of this church since I passed by it regularly but had no clue of the type of services being offered within. I remember sitting in the basement hall of this church with my friends. I don't recall if my friends were members of this church, but I do recall how comfortable they were with what was being asked of us. I wasn't. In order to belong to this camp and, in my mind, in order for me to stay with my friends, we were required to publicly welcome the Lord and renounce Satan. Praying, for me, had always happened silently within a quiet atmosphere of peace. I was in a personal battle between my beliefs and my wants. My wants won. I wanted friends, and at that time I believed I had to become someone else to maintain these particular friends.

So I prayed out loud and, being one who by then could easily speak in front of others, sounded believable. That skill helped me in creating friendships with those who were different from me but also created the confusion of who I had to be in order to have friends. That battle between who I was and who I wanted to be resulted in accumulating friends of various interests but being unable to sustain those friendships.

As I reached my teenage years, my need to be part of an "in" crowd was high, and I spent considerable time focussed on those who maintained contact with me. I was the entertainer. I could play the piano without needing sheet music. I was the one who had a car accessible for my friends for rides to school or to attend parties. I rarely drank alcohol, which was a bonus to others, and so became the token designated driver of the group. I was focussed on the now and didn't look past what was being seen on the surface.

Many of my high school friends were raised on farms, and we often congregated amongst isolated nooks and crannies in back fields outside of the city. For the majority of the week-days, we would be planning where the weekend parties would be. I always felt included, and even though I wasn't dating or in a relationship I did not question my status as any different to others. I was a companion to the females and a buddy to the males.

It became apparent one night after a few years of following this group how fragile these friendships were. This specific gathering was being held north of the city, and again I felt total acceptance, with my friends making sure I was attending. But it dawned on me that perhaps my popularity was due to the access I had to my family's car. On the way to the party my car was full. On the way home I was driving alone. Well, I wasn't actually alone. The two couples that had travelled with me were crammed in the back seat making out all the way home. It was one of those pitiful times when I felt isolated and so very different.

During my university years, many of the people I had maintained contact with as friends from my teenage years were connecting with their life partners and planning weddings. I thought of nothing but excitement when asked repeatedly to man a guest table at a wedding reception. Other female friends were designated as bridesmaids, but I really didn't notice the different status I was given, nor did I feel excluded. I was present for all preparations and celebrations.

A significant moment for me came when my brother Greg was getting married. Of the four sisters in my family, I regarded myself the closest to this new female member of our family. Greg's fiancée and I were close in age and hung out, spending occasional time together beyond the common family occasions when Greg was present. At least, I perceived that I was closest. Maybe being close had no direct relationship with who was asked to be part of the wedding party?

For this wedding, four of the six possible siblings on my side of the family were part of the wedding party. Allison and I were the only ones excluded. Allison had been living away from the family for over ten years, and I could understand why she was not included. I believed at the time I was excluded because I was not worthy enough to be included. To me, I should have tried harder to be a better friend.

Once I realized that my role was once again outside the inner circle, my understandings were two-fold. I questioned my perception of friendship and started wondering whether the close relationships I felt were in fact only within my view. Was I actually someone with whom people felt obligated to devote time? The second was blame. The inner anger was directed at me for not being of average height and thinking that it was my physical deformities that created these barriers from normalcy.

Continuing into my twenties and thirties, there were similar occurrences with various family and friends that only helped to confirm my perception that I was not worthy enough to stand up and be a formal witness at important celebrations of life. Each time, I would console myself with the secondary tasks that were granted to me and masked the hurt inside.

While writing this particular line about friendship in a poem so many years ago, I was struggling a lot with what friendship meant for me. My friends from my childhood were long gone, with the exception of one who was still studying in the city I had moved from. Others I spent considerable time with as a teenager were distant and heading off into various journeys of their own. The friends I met in university were focussed on establishing their own careers and personal lives within their communities.

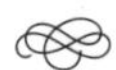

Acquiring my first professional job as a teacher was a challenge. I was met with numerous refusals, especially after the interview stage when employers would have had an opportunity to actually meet me. That year, I was one of thirty-two students graduating from our university who were specialized in my particular training, and I had assumed acquiring a job would be a simple process. At that time, the need for trained special education teachers in schools in our province was high. The majority of my peers were quickly hired by the larger communities prior to the May convocation ceremony, but I remained unemployed and started questioning the chances of success.

I started to apply to smaller communities of which I had no knowledge of or interest in. A bevy of resumes and applications were sent out, and while I received great notice and invitations to attend interviews, I was not succeeding in my quest to become an employed teacher. I mistakenly assumed that my university records did not impress others or my interview skills were lacking.

It was only after a director of a school division, without thought or compassion, explained his reluctance in hiring me that I understood the reality. This individual said his board's denial in hiring me was due to their concern of how I would cope with the "taller-than-me students" I would encounter. Well, those taller than me included anyone who was in grade one or beyond. So in his eyes, I was doomed for failure in my quest for any employment in teaching.

Fortunately, I ignored his concerns and kept on applying, believing someone would take a chance. It was a quiet community in the southeast corner of our province that took that chance. It really didn't matter that they were most desperate, and that I was probably the only qualified applicant – I obtained employment.

I accepted my first teaching position and began living in a new community, for the first time totally independent from family. This town was set near potash mines with about thirty-four hundred people living in or around the community. This was also a large farming area and the majority of students were bussed to the schools.

I was assigned to work part-time in each of the two

elementary schools of that community. My position was to work with students with learning concerns, and as well, work with the teachers who were responsible for these students. A classroom teacher's role can be an isolated one in terms of the amount of daily connections they have with other adults. My role in special education was the exact opposite. I was in daily contact with my colleagues within my schools and soon started establishing friendships within and beyond the school setting.

While I was missing those who knew me and brought me comfort, I was celebrating true independence. I could be me without anyone reminding me who I should be. For the first time, I was living in my own home without other family members, and could decide for myself how my furniture and personal items would be placed. I could leave my step stools anywhere and not worry about who was going to trip over them.

I showed great confidence as a beginning teacher and felt my teaching role was believable and trusted. I didn't waver in my decisions and seemed to have a great instinct in knowing what programs and supports were needed for students. At one point, one of my colleagues asked me how long I had been teaching. There was great surprise in learning that this was my first year. Many had assumed I had been teaching for at least ten years, a respectful compliment.

Teaching in this community required our professional staff to travel to larger cities to receive professional development training. While my colleagues and I were serious and attentive during the day, our evenings were more relaxed. One of the traditions while staying in hotels during teacher conferences was to play tricks on each other. This especially happened to the newbies of the group. I was sharing a room with another young teacher and was comfortable enough with the room to experience uninterrupted sleep the first night we were there. The next morning my friends kept on asking me how I had slept, and I was puzzled by their great interest in my sleeping habits. By the end of the sessions that day I found out the reason for their interest. My colleagues had short sheeted my bed … but I hadn't noticed.

Folding the bottom sheet halfway across the bed so that this sheet also becomes the top sheet is usually very evident when you climb into bed and try to extend your legs. It is a harmless joke requiring the recipient of the humour to strip the bed and remake it if they want to sleep in comfort. For me, while I recalled the sheets being awfully tight around my feet, I had no idea the sheet I was lying between had been folded in half.

Living alone in this new town provided me occasions to become acquainted with many individuals. My lifelong fascination and connection with friends who are years older than me was initiated in this community. I was fortunate to work with a teacher as she was finishing her career after forty years of service. Yana had been raised to and continued to respect the Doukhobor religious traditions of her Russian ancestors. I was fascinated with her home and often visited her and her husband on their farm. Yana's house was a traditional mud house, which was a common sight on the prairies a hundred years ago. She had the gift of storytelling, and I would sit for hours listening to the tales of her past.

There was another colleague who became a close friend, and we have remained in contact since that time. Lynn was one of those kind and soft individuals who it only made sense would be teaching grade-one students for the majority of her career. Lynn introduced me to her family members who were living in a nearby community and also encouraged me to get involved as a leader in a girls' organization similar to the Brownie troop I had belonged to so many years ago. Lynn included me on many social occasions and, through her, I met a couple who inspired this particular line from the poem.

Sitting on the sidelines observing intimate relationships between couples, I have always been fascinated with those who were well matched and expressed their love in front of others. The ones who were comfortable and secure in their connection also seemed to be comfortable in welcoming single individuals into their circle without hesitation. I was and still am friends to both such partners and not just a friend to one or the other. This couple I got to know back then was just that. I could talk to either one with comfort.

For the first year and part of my second year in this town, I was busy with friends and activities. This community was modest and more isolated than what I was used to, but I felt very involved and an integral part of the school and beyond. Close to my upcoming second pre-Christmas celebrations I would be participating in with this community, it was announced by this favourite couple of mine that the husband had been transferred, and they would be moving out of province at the beginning of the New Year.

My community of friends started making plans for a farewell celebration. With my take-charge organizing abilities, I started conversing with others about possible venues where we could hold this celebration. To my amazement, someone informed me bluntly that the celebration would be couples only.

I was appalled. It was the 1980s, not the 1950s. I was hurt by their intentions and further amazed when not one of the other included couples pointed out the rude exclusion of the single friends to this event. It was one of the first times when my single status, not my height, was measuring my acceptance with others, and I didn't know how to fix it.

That particular couple I had connected to did move, and I continued living within this town until the end of that same school year. As I was leaving the community, I was presented with a farewell gift. It was a framed collection of pictures highlighting different images including an aerial picture of the town and photos of the schools. Also included was a photo of the special couple I had gotten to know and respect. The irony was the print of the couple was included within a group picture that someone had captured at their "couples only" farewell dinner. I kept that frame for years as a reminder of the risk of wanting to be close.

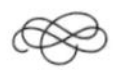

The struggle to figure out and sustain friendships has been similar to my yearning to learn to golf. Many of my female teaching friends in my home community years later would hustle out of school every Tuesday in the fall and spring to get on the golf course. They would return the next day and talk about their fun times. I wanted so much to be part of that fun.

One spring, I approached the resident golf pro and asked him how I could play golf. He was excited to take on this challenge and eagerly cut down some used golf clubs for me to learn the game. Soon afterwards, I was attending swing lessons and found myself practicing hitting balls straight down the fairway. I had always loved the mini-golf games we would play at the local resort town near our cabin, but now felt especially important that I had my own "real" golf clubs and could join my friends in an activity of common interest. Within a year, the golf pro arranged to have a set of custom clubs made for me, and I felt ready to join the others in this pastime.

Those who are kind and welcoming will invite me to play golf with them once, but as I have a limited driving ability these invitations are rarely repeated. While I can brag that my longest drive was about a hundred yards, my average drive down the fairway was sixty yards. Let's just say I never lost a ball. But I did lose golf partners. Waiting for me to get the golf ball to the green required patience and thick skin, as other golfers piled up behind us waiting for our group to move on. I continued to golf elsewhere, though, usually finding the shorter Par 3 courses that were better suited to my abilities. Gradually, I walked away from golf and used my spine issues as an excuse for not playing. My friendships with others are similar to my journey with golf. As with the golf games I wanted to play, I found it easier in my friendships to walk away rather than speak the truth of what I perceived within friendships with others.

I also started noticing a pattern with some friends and family members that the time they sought contact with me – who was single and without children – was dependent upon the present age of their children. The amount of attention and contact decreased when newborns and infants were part of their lives. The amount of attention increased when their offspring were teenagers or young adults busy in their own lives. This cycle repeated once again as grandchildren became part of their family. It was only natural this cycle occurred, but as the recipient of the cycled friendship, it was hard to adjust to these changes and expectations. Once acknowledged, I could understand and respect this cycle.

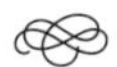

I know so many people or, more so, so many people know me. Many greet me by name as if we have shared experiences together, and I will have no clue of their identity. I have questioned my memory at times until I realized that the person conversing with me is actually a total stranger who has had access to my story. The attention I received from others because I was so physically different at times confused my perception of who my friends were. If someone was interested in getting to know me, I was never sure if that interest was for notoriety or true interest. I had and still have friends who call me a friend to others because of the attention this creates for them and the unique vignettes of my life they are able to share with others. I occasionally have difficulty trusting that it is my personal self that creates interest and not my different body shape. Great interest can be easily misinterpreted. A person showing care and attention may be just someone who is very kind with a mission, but I would read more into that interest. The perception of friendship and connecting with others has been, at times, an image. My images have been influenced by the way people perceived and treated me.

I have had numerous opportunities in acquiring friends, and

from this stands out one particular group of people who have taught me a lot about life. My family members, while I was growing up, were game players. There were decks of cards left on the kitchen table for easy access to a game of solitaire or fish. Crib boards and mind puzzle games were common items on the coffee table. Many times after a meal some of us would initiate a card or board game at the dining room table. I became addicted to game playing at a very young age and celebrated when someone else wanted to initiate a game. As I emerged into adulthood, many around me viewed playing games as a childhood practice and as my family members and friends got older they would show little interest in playing. That urge to play games never lessened for me, and I was so pleased when I discovered other adults who felt the same way.

There is one group in particular whom I call my "little old ladies." I have been friends with these older persons for a long time and have remained friends until their passing. These friendships started within my church many years ago when card parties were scheduled as a social one evening each week. I even purchased my existing home from the family of one of these friends. Most of these older friends were widows, but there were a few exceptions. We began getting to know each other at these gatherings and continued the tradition of playing games in each other's homes after the church discontinued that specific activity. Most members of this group were in their seventies when I first began to know them.

For a long while there was a tradition of the little old ladies gathering at a local Chinese food restaurant and then heading off to someone's home afterward for game playing. The person hosting the event would always provide the required pots of English tea with the milk poured into the cups before the tea. Glasses of cold water were always present for me and another member. At the end of the evening, a dessert was offered for consumption and no one declined.

While I feel everyone in this special group have all been faithful friends to me throughout the years, I have certainly challenged their faith in my friendship. I was the only one working full time and on many occasions felt too busy to meet with them. These friends would go out of their way to change the date and time of their next card game to fit my needs. There were a couple of occasions when I would forget to attend an expected supper and come home from work to find messages on my home phone with them worrying about me. My apologies in forgetting about an event were never accepted, and they always understood and forgave how "busy" I was. Their strong bond of friendship was a gift to me and taught me one of my most important lessons of forgiveness in life.

This lesson happened the same year Dad had passed, and I was still grieving months after he had gone. That fall, I decided I wanted to put together an updated video montage of pictures of Dad with music that also included the video that Dad and I had made those many years ago. I was using the school secretary's computer to create this video production and worked hours each night, ignoring other obligations and responsibilities. My deadline was to complete the project by Christmastime in order to gift my family members with this special remembrance.

Close to the holiday season, I hosted a supper and card night for my little old ladies. I was so proud of what I had completed for my family and wanted to share a preview of my video with these friends. I didn't ask, but instead started the video, then turned to watch those viewing the pictures. Their expressions were not what I was expecting. They were captured prisoners watching something not of their choice.

I was so wrapped up in my grieving process and my need to heal through this video project that I did not account for their current lives. Sitting watching this video was a couple who had lost one of their adult children to cancer only a month before Dad had passed. Sitting there was a recent widow who had lost her husband a month after Dad passed. The others who had been widows for a long while also could feel the uncomfortable tension in the room. The video, while full of visual pictures of happiness, included music of gloom and reflection. It was a theme of saying farewell and totally inappropriate to be shown to those who were still within their own period of mourning.

I quickly apologized but realized the reality of not being able to take that one mistake back. I thought I had damaged an important friendship and went silent, letting them back away. But these people, who walked the faith, did something totally different. Within weeks of that meal, I was invited out again and in the middle of the restaurant was presented with a gift thanking me for showing them the video. I was confused then realized how important these people were to me and how important I was to them. A few of these friends from years back are still part of my life. We meet occasionally, and I am heartbroken when another one passes. At each passing, I am so thankful for the opportunities I have had with them and continue to cherish the lessons they have taught me.

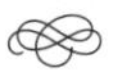

I could name many, but there is one friend in particular who has been there throughout the majority of my years of teaching and beyond. Emma Lee and I met after I had been transferred from one elementary school to another. I was looking forward to working at this new school for many reasons, including having an opportunity to be a classroom teacher. My mother was a grade-one classroom teacher years before at the same school. I was also hoping for the move in order to continue my relationship with my current principal. When I found out that he was being transferred, I soon after made a request to follow him and his leadership.

Emma Lee was not only a teacher, but also a parent of this new school. I was grateful to be a classroom teacher to both of her children. I remember Emma being one of the first to welcome me. She generously shared professional materials and advice as I coped with being a classroom teacher for the first time in my career. We soon became close friends and colleagues and I began to spend time with her family outside of the school day.

Emma Lee and I at some point in our relationship decided we should join the local adult community band. I am not sure why. I wanted to be part of a band, though reluctantly, considering my far-off memories of playing in a classroom band years ago in junior high school. During those pre-teen years I tried to avoid being singled out or given extra attention. Unfortunately, considerable attention and focus was placed on me as the music teacher those years ago tried to figure out which instrument I would be able to play. My short arm length limited my ability to play the typical "girl" instruments such as the flute or clarinet. Trumpets, saxophones and obviously the trombone were also taken off the list. I was assigned the French horn and reluctantly dragged this large, heavy, brass instrument home each week to practice during the three years while attending that school.

Decades later, when Emma and I arrived for our first band practice, similar discussions focussed on which instrument I would be capable of playing. Time for me to flee. It took Emma a few more years of persuasion to get me to return to the band hall and try again. In the meantime, the band director had been doing some investigating and offered a suggestion that I consider purchasing and playing a curved soprano saxophone. I was acquainted with what a straight soprano saxophone looked like but never knew that the curved shape similar to an alto or tenor saxophone was possible in a size suitable for my arm length.

Playing the soprano saxophone has opened many new doors including working on improving my reluctance to play alongside other musicians. In order to learn to play this instrument well I had to make an effort to practice regularly to further develop skills. There are times when I forget to practice or have been too engaged doing other activities. It takes time and commitment to play a musical instrument with talent. Friendships, such as the one I have with Emma Lee, require similar devotion and time. Patience, understanding and trust also contribute to the success of sustaining lasting friendships.

I have come to understand that the words I wrote so long ago about comfort and lies that I believe referred to my friends were instead written about me. I was aware that my friends were not really sharing with me their true feelings and thoughts, but perhaps I was not providing them invitation or opportunity to do so. I had masked so many of my hurts and fears that I thought sharing my honest views would break apart friendships. My need to be the same at times hindered the true potential relationship of my friends. While I sought comfort from others, I did not always have the ability to give back comfort to others while I was coping with who I was. I needed to focus on me to help sustain me. I had no idea then that giving to others was what I needed for me to be me.

I have come to realize that it is our current life experiences that define who our current set of friends are. It is only rational that friends who gather together to ski, to dance or engage in other physical activities that I am not able to complete would be more distant to me than those with whom I share common experiences. It is understandable that those who, like me, are single or not raising children, would be attracted to each other as friends. Those who we are currently occupied with in our daily activities become the friends, at that specific moment, who are the most important to us.

My need to sustain existing friendships was my need, and while I recognized that these friends close to me would always be near, the degree of contact and amount of sharing would naturally change as our experiences changed. One of my favourite times has been when a friendship has grown apart but when we do have the opportunity to meet again we both realized distance and time were not important. The conversations continued as if we had spoken yesterday. It was with these friends that I could be certain that a connection would always be there and we would have each other's support forever.

It wasn't until years later when a colleague I was working with shared a particular piece of writing with me that I truly understood what my role as a friend could be. It is written by Marianne Williamson, from her book *A Return to Love.*[9] The passage starts with the words, "Our deepest fear is not that we are inadequate. Our deepest fear is that we are powerful beyond measure. It is our light, not our darkness that most frightens us." Those words changed my perception and seemed to give me permission to share my light with others.

My relationships with friends remain important for me. I look forward to seeing others, but also am comfortable staying at home and being alone. I love being included in their celebrations and love including them in mine. My friends are my family, my colleagues and the ones who I trust and admire. My friends are a reflection of me.

The celebration of friends, their diversity and care

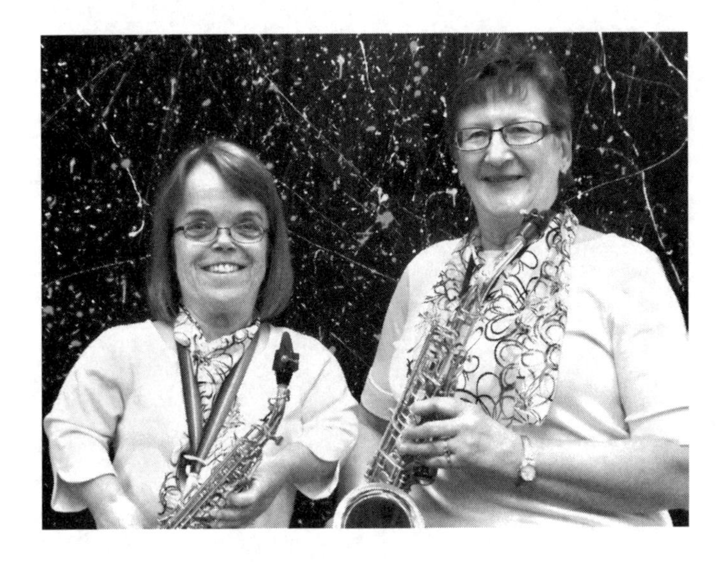

Emma Lee and I after playing a saxophone duet at a band concert.

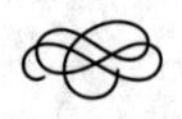

Chapter 6

The pain of a stranger, the names, the eyes, the degradation

A lot of my memories of encountering strangers while growing up and during my early adult years were centred on answers to one question: "How are they going to react?" Because my family did not hide me or restrict me from wandering around my community, there were many times when I would go walking or exploring on my own. It was inevitable I would meet up with someone who did not know me, and I could expect a range of reactions. As one who likes to categorize, it is easy for me to slot those responses into tight boxes.

Most noticeable were those who seemed to have no social filters or boundaries; in other words, just plain rude. Strangers would stop, look a second time and then react. What was it about being a Little Person that gave strangers permission to strike out in rudeness and aggression? Most often they were at a distance that required them to yell their response. I could hear it blocks away … "Hey, Midget!" "There's a midget!" "Look, a midget!" If only they would say it once and then walk on, I would have an opportunity to ignore them. But rarely did they walk on. Usually, if it was said in this aggressive manner, the person saying it wasn't alone. I was always alone. Most of the time, a physical encounter was going to be the outcome. I was never sure whether these individuals wanted to harm me, but most of them felt comfortable enough in approaching me to continue their verbal attacks right up to my face. This was where my choices of responses would need to kick in.

I could ignore it and pretend I couldn't hear what was being said. This skill has become well mastered. I could stop and attempt to stare them down, hoping for some realization of their inappropriate words. I could interrupt their prattle of name-calling and educate them on the proper decorum of respectful language related to Little People. I could assimilate the same language usage and tone they were expressing and create my own version of truth in return, most often including every epithet within my vocabulary. Or I could flee.

Fleeing was my preferable mode, but obviously the least effective. I naturally didn't move as fast, and would soon have to use another solution. My most memorable attempt of fleeing happened in a local department store during my early years of teaching.

I was in the ladies' clothing section searching for "professional" outfits for teaching. Purchasing clothing has never been one of my favourite chores for many reasons, including the need to reach up to high racks to select items to try on. But on that particular day, those racks filled with clothing came in handy. I was examining an item of clothing when a lady and her son approached me, with the lady saying loudly, "Come here, honey, come and look at the midget." I looked over at the two and observed a tall, skinny, middle-aged woman dragging a young, reluctant, apprehensive child. This child was fearful of me and of what his mother was asking him to do.

I began weaving in and out of the clothing racks, masking my body from them, and hoping they would get the message that I was not interested in continuing this interaction. No such luck. As I continued to weave, so did the mother, successfully dragging her child behind her and continuing her loud pleas to her child of the importance of examining me. This had to stop. I was running out of clothing racks to circle around. I held my ground, waited for her to catch up, and then blasted her with harsh words, pointing out her obvious rudeness. There was no apology, which didn't surprise me. Instead, a quiet slinking away by both of them occurred.

I have always hated having to do this in front of children, especially a child with whom I can identify. That child was as scared as I was from this encounter and now, with my aggressive words, was probably even more fearful of future encounters with people who are different. This leads to my second classification of encounters with strangers: those who are scared.

How many people can say they have the ability to elicit a cry from a child just by walking towards them? I am usually able to determine this level of fear just by observing a person's eyes. It is most often a child under the age of six or seven who experiences this extreme reaction of fear, but I have also witnessed adults who have displayed a similar response.

For the frightened child, the outcome of whether the encounter resulted in a full-blown meltdown of emotion and fear or the encounter resulted in something better was usually dependent upon the adults who were with the child. I have been witness to numerous potential injuries of children who have been forcibly pulled away from my presence by parents abruptly yanking their child's arms and directing them on another path. Parents have covered the eyes of children as I am passing in order for them to quit staring. Parents have shut down their child's natural curiosity when they ask out loud why I am small, thus providing for that child the interpretation that getting to know about me is not appropriate. My favourite is when parents feel they are the experts and start explaining to the child, while in front of me, the reason for my disfigurement. The "drinking too much coffee" explanation has been used many times.

Children are naturally inquisitive and when they encounter something different they want to investigate. They are hesitant, they are careful, but if they have been raised in an environment of encouragement, their interaction with someone like me for the first time is usually a positive one.

No sane person wants to instill fear in anybody else, and for me to do so just by standing in front of a child who does not comprehend my differences continues to be one of the greatest heartaches I have encountered. Very young toddlers have no fear, but also have no idea that I am an adult. They greet me as one of their own and invite me to play with them. I love that. The parent who trusts that I will not harm their child will quietly supervise the interaction this child and I are having.

With the recent interest in portraying dwarves in various reality TV shows, the awareness of LPs is increasing and the isolation of being a private Little Person is disappearing. All aspects of being a dwarf, including intimate and emotional aspects of being different, are being shared as they are played out in these "celebrities'" lives. Some doors of understanding from these shows have been opened, but followers of these shows forget they are watching just a show of entertainment. Strangers have always been making comments that are invasive and judgmental in nature. Now they are just more personal. I have collected too many to include, but here are some of the doozies:

> "How's the weather down there?"
> "Can I pick you up?"
> "I feel so sorry for you because I am tall and you aren't."
> "Can I take your picture?"
> "You are so cute."
> "Can she talk?"
> "I so enjoy watching your show."
> "Hey, short stuff."

My favourite and quite common reaction when someone sees me for the first time is the exclamation, "Whoa!" I'm not a horse and I definitely do not plan to stop for you. It is a natural expression that you know the person didn't mean to say, but their social filters were not ready for the sight of me. Some apologize, some then ignore me as we walk by but others, whose social filters were never fully developed, continue with additional explanative comments making sure others around them can hear as well.

I have become very proficient at not acknowledging the stares, the gestures and the rudeness of others. I am always aware of the attention, but most times choose not to acknowledge it. Many of my family members have witnessed those staring running into doorways, or tripping over objects, as their eyes have remained focussed on me. If I am me and comfortable being me, I rarely "see" those mishaps and opportunities for humour.

Other siblings have had similar situations, but my sister Ivory has been present for those majorities of times when strangers have approached me. Ivory has had to point to me when waiters are asking her what I want to eat in a restaurant. She has had to patiently wait beside me while young children approach and unexpectedly start engaging in play conversation with me. Ivory has had to master the "get out of her face" look to others who are staring or wanting to grab my attention. She at times has also been a physical barrier between that somewhat scary stranger and me.

My family members and friends seem more upset with rude people than I am. My siblings who live near me seem to catch the majority of comments, gestures or actions that are being directed to me when I have not noticed. It's funny, but it's not, that even those who I have known for the majority of my life will think that making a joke about my height in public is acceptable.

Those close to me can be vigilant and have actually written letters or made phone calls if they feel that attempts of humour that were actually hurtful have been directed my way. I prefer running away from the uncomfortable. I prefer letting it go. But at times, I have had to stop and allow those who absorb the intended hurt beside me to react with their own preference.

There was one incident where the master of ceremonies at a very large event was repeatedly asking me to stand up to be recognized. I was standing. The emcee's third or fourth repetition of the request, and attempt of humour, was turning from a slight agitation of the request to members in the room becoming enraged with this obvious faux pas of how to treat Little People. If you really want to know what it is like to be a Little Person, you need to realize that we never stand up and we never sit down in the average person world. In this world of height differences, for me to stand up from an adult-size chair usually involves me having to jump down. For me to sit down on a chair that is made for an average person, I have to climb up. My view or perception of what I can see standing down and sitting up is also opposite to the norm.

I am no different. There are moments in my life when I have behaved harshly or been rude to others. I have learned, though, that the opportunity to repair that uncomfortable moment is only possible at that point of time. It is difficult to go back and make amends, and this difficulty increases in proportion to the time elapsed. Our relationships with each other change with each difficult moment that has been ignored.

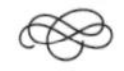

Being the recipient of constant rudeness has been fairly easy to cope with; being frightened has not. I have encountered scary relationships where the person involved becomes obsessed with my differences. Those people want to pet me or hug me upon immediate contact. Some invade my personal space and try to pick me up or crowd me into a corner to examine me. They have a need to physically verify my existence. They are touchers who have few or no filters of consciousness. The farther these people are from general civilization, the higher degree of creepiness is expressed. Some ask permission to carry out an action that involves an invasion of my personal space, and I am forced to protect my rights and privacy and voice a strong no.

At the time of writing the line about strangers in the poem, I was living in an apartment building while teaching. I had met a few of the habitants, but the majority of those residing in my building were potash mine employees who worked different time shifts. One Sunday afternoon, I was baking and had run out of a dry ingredient. I didn't want to go out in the cold weather and decided to knock on doors down my hallway to see if a neighbour could rescue me.

Across the hall from me lived a single young man who was probably close to my age. I knocked on his door and when he answered asked him whether he had the baking ingredient I was missing. Other than knowing he was working at the local mine, I hadn't met him before. It was a short conversation. I didn't get my needed item and had to run to the store instead. That one impulsive action of knocking on his door set forth a series of strange incidents.

For the next little while, this neighbour would knock on my apartment door and strike up conversations that I saw as friendly interest. I didn't invite him in, but had a series of conversations in the hallway for the next few weeks. I can't recall the exact reason I started withdrawing from the conversations, but I was picking up that maybe this person had some issues I should avoid. I became very busy when we passed by and started to limit the conversations to a friendly hello.

The distance I created angered him, and I soon started receiving very scary, dark drawings slipped under my door during the middle of the night. I was so disgusted by what was being depicted in those drawings that I actually immediately destroyed them. I didn't show them to anyone. I didn't complain to anyone. Instead, I holed up in my apartment, deciding that to socially reach out to others in the building was not a healthy choice. This neighbour eventually was evicted from the building after accidentally setting his kitchen on fire while passed out.

A different scary encounter occurred during a cruise vacation a few years later. I decided I needed to prove my independent status as an adult and booked a Christmas holiday alone on a cruise ship that would be travelling through the Panama Canal. I had been on a cruise ship with some of my family previously to this trip and felt confident that staff on board could solve any challenges I encountered.

For the majority of this ten-day cruise I was alone but was not feeling alone. Our ship had just passed through the Panama Canal and passengers were recovering from the New Year's celebrations the crew had hosted for the past two days. We were anchored off the San Blas Islands, and passengers were encouraged to disembark and wander around the Native community. I walked along the main streets where vendors were selling their crafts to interested passengers and decided to explore a side street off the main path. I came across a group of Natives who resided there.

I had already noticed that these people were very short, with most of the adults being less than five feet tall. Once they saw me, they swarmed around me and started touching and patting me, speaking in an unknown language. There were no cruise ship officials nearby and my only thought was to get away as quickly as I could. It took some doing and a lot of fast walking, but I soon made it back to the dock and was so pleased to be amongst familiar faces.

I look back now and realize that they meant no harm but were interested in my similarities to them. My past is what alarmed me the most. Having been chased and followed by others so many times, I reverted to my 'panic, must flee' mode and didn't recognize those peoples' natural interest in someone who was of similar height.

With the increased access to digital photography devices it has been the intrusive picture-takers that have recently invaded my space. Some would seek permission to take a photo of me and were always surprised when I said no. There were others who didn't ask. If I was suspicious and turned around as I was walking by, I usually saw a device aimed at me. It also happened when walking towards them. Suddenly, a device was pulled out, and they were rapt in viewing the device's screen. The chances of just having a photo or video taken of me were relatively high. If I were in a certain mood and not on a schedule, I would whip out my own device and pretend to take their picture in return. Their embarrassed expressions and quick departure confirmed my suspicions.

The accessibility of counselling to help relieve all my anxieties about encountering strangers was possible, but I often joked I would probably need to hire a professional full time. When tall males with darker hair approached me for the first time, a quiver of fear sometimes made itself know as I remembered my grade three experience. Consciously, I knew I was safe, but I still had trouble trusting that I was safe.

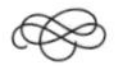

For more than thirty years, I have been an ambassador teaching children about skeletal dysplasia and differences, particularly in newly assigned schools. There was a pattern I would follow when moving into a new school. For the first two days of classes, I would make sure I was visible, volunteering for extra playground supervision, so the entire student body would have an opportunity to see me. The students would return to school the next day, some armed with inaccurate knowledge of who I was. Some were brave and started testing my boundaries of discipline right away with their name-calling. Some were scared stiff and would become a part of the wall as much as they could while I walked past them. By the third day, most students had noticed me, and many were asking me inane questions or sharing outrageous comments. Those words were not their own; those words were what their parents were saying to them once they had heard about me. It was at that point that I knew it was time for the "Me" lessons.

When orienting children to dwarfism and specifically the

topic of achondroplasia, I initiated lessons discussing the terms "same" and "different." I began by comparing myself with another adult present in the classroom. Children would then begin to notice the more "normal" details of me as an adult such as the watch I was wearing or the glasses on my face. To explain my dwarfism, I used simple drawings showing how a "normal" bone in an arm or leg grows and contrasting those drawings to others showing how bones in people with achondroplasia grow. My bones may have lengthened a bit since birth; however, most of the bone growth happened in a horizontal manner. I described the shape of the end of each bone in my arms or legs as a mushroom. Children could relate to those types of simple comparisons.

By the end of the lesson, most younger children were more interested in how big the bed I slept in was, or if I drove a car. Consistently, the minute I disclosed I wore size 12 children shoes, the younger students would begin taking off their shoes checking what size shoes they wore. Sometimes the lesson ended with an impromptu field trip to view the workings of the hand control in my car.

For older students, lessons included thoughtful discussions about open acceptance of all differences and how the continuation of prejudice among us can hurt. For each new school placement, the series of lessons was successful, and after I waited through the period of a "celebrity" status to settle down I could carry out my duties with the focus on teaching.

As a teacher, my relationship with children was unique, and students would seek out my attention for many reasons. Some would seek me out because they themselves were encountering their own challenges in life and felt a kinship to me. They seemed to appreciate the counselling I could provide in helping them resolve their challenges. Others were fascinated with my differences. I felt like I was their new toy or interest and would wait for that attention to wane. Others, I just felt, believed in my abilities and trusted me as a mentor to their learning.

I celebrated throughout my last year of teaching. I celebrated that I had made it. I was qualified to retire while still teaching, without any pension penalties. When I was first diagnosed in my forties with my spinal conditions, I had met with the STF and school board representatives asking what supports I could possibly receive if it was decided I could no longer work as a teacher. I was assured that my expected income would be supported if a full-time medical leave became necessary.

There were many discussions for the next fifteen years or so about what supports or accommodations I needed from my employers and health plan. At no point did I have to consider stopping my career and possibly spending extended years on a medical disability until I qualified for retirement. It was close, though, with the last few years of teaching requiring me to take a long-term half-time medical leave, which resulted in draining my sick leave allowance.

An ironic situation occurred on my last official day as an employed teacher. On the last momentous day of reaching retirement and still being active as a part-time teacher, I decided to go visit colleagues at a nearby school to wish them a happy summer. I had parked my car in the teacher's parking lot and was walking toward the front entrance of the school when a voice from the playground area yelled out, "Hey, midget."

Long ago, someone pointed out to me that my presence in a school was a lifelong lesson to students just by me being there. Whenever I became frustrated or angry at situations within my role as a teacher this shared observation helped remind me that I had bigger and greater things to accomplish, including educating strangers about differences. That student, who did not know me, on my last official day of work, helped me realize two things. One, there would always be individuals needing to be taught manners. Two, it didn't matter how many schools I worked in or how long I taught, I would always be yelled at.

Since I have taught close to thirty years in my own community it has been very common for strangers to approach me who really were not strangers. Former students from various schools I had worked in have made special efforts to approach and initiate a conversation with me. These tall grownups, whose features seemed vaguely familiar were, and still are, always so pleased to greet me even though I was usually standing there having no idea of their identity. I was elated for the times when they mentioned their name and I could think of the exact class and year I had taught them. For some, additional probing for more data helped in my recollection of that individual.

In every encounter with a former student, I was left with a feeling of accomplishment. Most conveyed the importance of what I had taught them, and I am humbly thankful that my efforts to encourage positive character traits and fine work habits influenced some part of their life. Some of these former students indicated I made an impact in their lives while others just by their positive, secure expressions and their accomplishments so far in life confirmed to me my belief that I did make a difference.

My interactions with strangers have improved, or the anxiety of dealing with rude persons has lessened, as compared to when I was a young adult. The eyes are still looking. The names volleyed my way are still thrown. The moments of degradation still occur. But how I react to those eyes, hear those words and experience the uncomfortable moments has changed.

I love being in a crowd of strangers. In my community, it is rare to come across someone who hasn't met me, heard about me or seen me in passing. Travelling gives me opportunities to interact with strangers, and I get to experience unique opportunities of connecting with someone for a short blip of time. Flying for hours in a plane, for example, is a venue that allows you a single time to interact with someone. The likelihood of meeting, once again, is nil. You have no history with these strangers; you have no expectations put upon you.

I know I am in a comfortable spot with a stranger when I am feeling equal in the conversation. It isn't one-sided with the person trying to sponge from me all facts and information about my differences in a limited time. It isn't when I am sensing I need to put on my showman's hat and entertain that frightened person so they will be comfortable in my presence. Instead, it is an exchange of dialogue that soon develops into something special for that moment of time. Usually, the stranger and I have discovered a common interest and will explore our differences within that interest. It is uncanny how strangers connect to others who are mirrors to them, and I so love those moments of realization when I have made another connection with one who is a reflection of me. Rarely do we make plans to extend this initial dialogue to another time. Instead, we part, and I am left with a full feeling of belief in what our world could be.

Sometimes strangers do become friends; sometimes friends become strangers. This is also true for our relationships between family and even those we love. At times, it is hard to distinguish the differences between family, friends and strangers. It is unfortunate when a relationship with a member of a family or a close friend distances to a degree of feeling like a stranger. For me, it is a fitting time to decide whether that relationship needs to be worked on or let go.

Our perceptions of relationships are changing continually. Sometimes we are close to those who should be important, and sometimes circumstances happen that interrupt those connections. In order to feel like myself, it is an awareness of who is joining me on my current journey, whose journey I am joining in on and whose journeys I am now needing to let go.

The interest of strangers, their acceptance and journeys

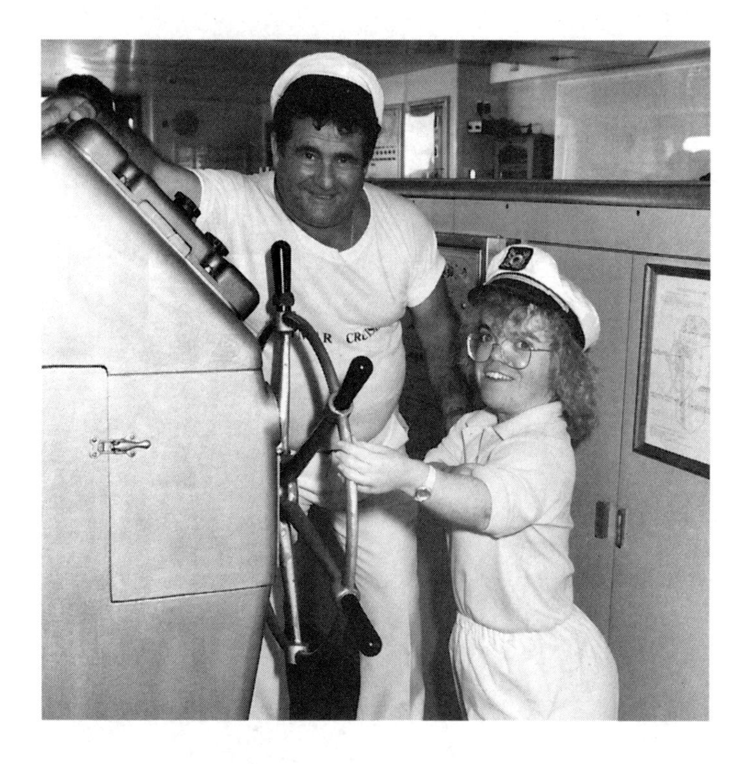

Steering the ship during an independent trip.

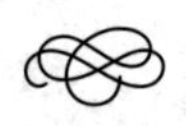

Chapter 7

The pain of the one I love, the obsessive giving to one who does not see

I believe that to write a memoir without disclosing your most embarrassing moments in life is leaving out who you really are. The private aspects of my life have been an area that I am reluctant to disclose, not only because of my own embarrassment, which is obvious, but also because of the potential of embarrassing others.

As a young child, I had become used to receiving attention from others, but the attention from males is what I craved the most. I viewed the females close to me as my caregivers and the males as my emotional supporters. I would seek my father's attention and the attention of my brothers, and it would be given. Any male relatives, especially my uncles, who visited us, seemed to be pleased to spend time with me, and I preferred their attention more so than the females in the crowd.

There were many neighbourhood friends who were males, and I thought nothing of hanging out with them as we explored our community. While I played with the typical Barbies and imaginary dress-up scenarios with my female friends, my preference was to be outside creating intriguing, investigative challenges that would miraculously be solved before suppertime. We were a mixed group in the neighbourhood who enjoyed the same type of play.

My interests changed during the years attending my junior high school, though. All of a sudden, boys became fascinating and cool. But it wasn't just the boys; it was also the younger male teachers who were very attractive. I was so normal, an emerging adolescent, female, and progressing into the turbulent emotional roller coaster of hormones. At the same time, I was becoming aware of my differences from others and starting to realize the impact of my dwarfism. I was a yo-yo, bouncing from one extreme emotional wall to another. It was at this time when I was introduced to romance, or what I thought was love.

During the summer months, Mom would pack up those of us who were not old enough to be working on the farm, and we would move to the lake. The stories of our times at the cabin could fill another book. It was a place to escape and relax. It was a place for me to hook up once a year with my lake friends. There were two friends in particular with whom I spent considerable time as an emerging teenager: Rachel, whose cabin was right next door to us, and Holly, who lived in one of the two palatial houses on top of the hill overlooking the lake.

Rachel was always already there when I arrived for the

summer. Her family drove across the province to reach our beach and planted themselves firmly there for the entire holiday. Rachel was a daredevil, always having plans for the day, which I would eagerly want to join in. She was also one of those friends with whom I never felt physically short. Rachel had her own medical issues to cope with, and looking back, I believe we were kindred spirits.

Holly, who lived in the palace on the hill, was also a summer immigrant arriving from a greater distance. She and her family would come to stay with her grandparents. Everything about her seemed physically perfect to me. Holly was tall, skinny and blonde with very cute features.

Holly introduced me to "love." Reading had always been a substantial part of our family's idle times, and there was a variety of reading materials on every surface in our home. I had no idea, until one particular summer, that one genre of fiction was being excluded from the choices given to me at home – romance.

Holly was a few years older than me and always carried a romance paperback around with her when I visited. One day, I picked up a book and started reading it. That was the beginning of a lifelong reading habit. That was and still is my drug, my escape. I could transfer myself into a storyline filled with romance and intrigue knowing that the outcome was always the same: love, acceptance and most importantly, happily ever after.

The obsession in seeking love as a teenager is normal. But my life has never been within the norm. My seeking love as a teenager definitely did not fit the standard "boy meets girl" scenario. I was receiving attention from strangers, attention from my friends, and attention from my family. I was also receiving attention from certain males who I believed I loved. Looking back, I probably should have had some sort of intervention or counselling. The two males who were the first to receive my obsession were kind, patient and probably very uncomfortable with my outpouring of emotion. They were also my teachers.

One teacher was my identity, the mirror of me. He was funny, he was engaging and he was also somewhat physically shorter than the other teachers in my junior high school. I look back now and realize I wanted to be like him in regard to his manner with others. I just had difficulty at that age differentiating between admiration and love. I believe I succeeded in absorbing a lot of his positive qualities as a teacher and ended up emulating him by sharing those qualities with my students.

The other teacher was my dream taken straight from the novels I had started reading. He was a young, sensitive professional who was teaching for the first time in a middle school. He taught me a few subjects, but my interest in him was heightened during a series of field trips where he relaxed his professional cloak and became buddies with the students. My interest in him was a quiet, sitting-on-the-sidelines type of obsession. I would find excuses to visit his classroom. My marks dramatically increased in his class in an effort to receive his attention.

The true, full-blown, off-tilt obsession came after this young teacher and his wife moved away from our community. I was heartbroken, emotional and irrationally devastated by his absence. I had already started to switch my focus and attention onto that second professional within my school, but then something happened. I learned that this first teacher had moved to a certain community on the other side of the province. I was determined to find out exactly where he had gone and planned to reach out to him.

I do not recall specifically how I succeeded in acquiring this person's personal contact information, but I did. This was way before the era of online digital information where one can easily access the Internet to make such inquiries. I obtained his address, and I wrote to him. The unfortunate thing is, he wrote back. My obsessive infatuation was confirmed. I knew he was married, and I believe at that time he was expecting his first child, but in my eyes he cared for me.

I remember taking the letter to school and telling everyone I had received a letter from this teacher. I don't think I ever admitted I was the one who wrote first. I would have had to explain how I "stalked" him to find where he had moved. It embarrasses me to remember how I continued writing to him, becoming more personal in my words and tone. I started addressing him by his first name and sharing my personal days with him.

I was so fortunate that I had selected for my obsession an individual who was kind but also a professional. As a teacher who has received these typical gestures of puppy love from adolescent students, I now appreciate how this particular teacher handled this uncomfortable situation. He quit responding. It took a few more letters on my part before I eventually figured out what the silence meant and I quit harassing him.

I continued to prefer spending time with males at social occasions, but really never returned to that irrational, aggressive obsession for the rest of my schooling. Instead, I found avenues that allowed me to interact with male teenagers without putting them into situations of discomfort.

One of my favourite experiences was when I started working as a cashier at our local hockey rink during my last two years of high school. The cashiers were required to be at the rink early to greet the first customer coming in, but would also have opportunity to talk to the players who were there ahead of the game. As employees, we would catch the third period of most games after our shift was completed. My knowledge of hockey increased, and I would sometimes find myself at school the following day sitting with the male members of my class talking about last night's game. Through these discussions, I became comfortable being amongst males my age.

My interests were so out of tune with what my female friends were discussing, like clothes, makeup and attending the next dance. To me, the idea of wearing makeup was foreign and shopping for clothing to me had always been an ongoing challenge. And dancing? Well, that's another chapter ...

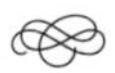

There are times in our lives when we are connected to a person and for some reason that person just knows you without explanation. You care for that person and know that you are cared for in return. We are fortunate when that happens to us. There was one male friend in particular who stands out. Unfortunately for my friend, my perception of feelings were so screwed up that he was the greatest victim of my silent obsession. This is a personal, intrusive story, which needed his permission to tell.

George became my friend when I was seven years old when we began walking to school together. George was two years younger than me and was a part of a family living across the street from us. While I was one of the youngest in my family, he was the oldest. I had six siblings; he would eventually be one of three.

His family was my second family, and often I would escape to his home. His mother was the mother I, at times, longed for. My mother, out of necessity and survival, often addressed my concerns with a business-like approach. George's mother was one who often included me in their family plans and would incessantly tell me wonderful things about myself. She still does.

George and I were close friends through our years of schooling yet did not have the need for continued contact with each other. He had his own set of friends closer to his age, and I had mine. When we eventually got together it was always just a continuation of a conversation that had seemed to start a minute ago. We shared everything important to us and when important decisions needed to be made we would seek each other out. I even recall spending endless amounts of time talking with George on the phone when we were steps away from walking over and sharing our thoughts in person.

George was my constant. My other friends came and went depending upon their particular interests, but George was always there. When I moved away for my university years, I greatly missed those conversations I seemed to need with George. I would come home on weekends, and my first quest was to connect with my friend. When change is created by distance or time, our perception of that relationship should also change, but not for me.

Rarely up until this time period did I compare myself to George's other friends. But now I saw myself to be the visitor in his home, more in the role of an observer. He or his family didn't change, I did. The ever-increasing number of female friends who were part of his life bothered me. While we continued to connect in the same manner as before, my need for more was making itself quietly known to me. My regard for him was changing, and I didn't have any previous experience to fall back on other than that of my obsessive attention with two former teachers.

George never changed in his regard for me, but my perception of his regard changed. He was, and always will be, a very kind person. He had this intent focus and attention on the person he was talking to, and you couldn't help but feel special in his presence. George loved life and sharing that love of life with others.

I am attracted to and will always prefer to be around those types of men. I seem to prefer to connect with men who are more passive. For whatever reason, I unrealistically started to believe that George and I would someday be life partners.

For the last two years of university, George had moved to the same city to start his own years of college, and I was in my glory. It didn't matter that I had already started seeing things within George that would define his natural preferences in relationships with others. I was with my buddy, my companion and kept my feelings for him to myself. Or at least I thought I did.

My brother Lyle recognized something. Instead of ignoring my obsession with George, which I assumed other siblings and friends clearly saw as well, he presented George with a gift. Lyle, without my knowledge or permission, took a few of the romance books, which I had piled into a corner by my bed, wrapped them and presented them to George. When George opened that gift in front of others during some sort of celebration, I was mortified. George was confused. George knew I read romances for fun and couldn't figure out why Lyle had given them to him. I look back and realize now that maybe Lyle's actions weren't directed to me, but maybe he was conveying his own message to George.

I remember the first time I saw another female friend hug George and the dawning realization of my "just a friend" status. It was during my last year of university, and while George and I were still friends, another person had joined us to form a triangle. It wasn't some evil person who had hugged George in my presence. It was my sister Ivory.

Ivory had moved to the city to start her own education and was part of the social outings whenever George was included. If I had thought rationally about it, George and Ivory had also attended high school together and were closer in age. I had been away from my hometown for two years attending university, so their friendship had had an opportunity to further develop. We were now a group of three going out for meals and watching movies together.

I was immaturely jealous of the activities George and Ivory could do, from which I felt excluded. Over the years, they would bike and even ski together. These were things I could not do or thought I could not do. As we moved from our educational years to our professional careers, George and I remained friends, but our friendship had now changed. I gradually gained recognition that my obsession with George was just that – my obsession. The line from the poem clearly acknowledges, "One who did not see." George did not see. He didn't have to.

When someone is raised to be kind and respectful to others they are not going to do anything that will embarrass others. I believed George did see some of my immature advances but chose to kindly ignore them. As young adults, a pattern formed between George and me of exchanging letters, phone calls and visits. Rarely did we continue that exchange of our true inner thoughts as we had once done as children and teenagers. I clung to what was and still cared for him but was not willing to admit to my perception of that care.

George had many opportunities for travel in his quest to further his career. I was disheartened when he moved away but this distance helped in creating more rational feelings. It's uncanny, but I would have these bouts of telepathic knowledge involving George, and I knew ahead of time when a contact or a visit from him was coming my way within a day's time.

George was handy because of his ever-increasing physical distance and his lack of presence in my community. Sometimes I would use the essence of George as a fodder for storytelling when questioned why I didn't have a boyfriend or husband. I would exaggerate my friendship with him into a more intimate relationship to distract others from my obvious single status. These instances only refuelled my reluctance to address the reality of what I needed to do with an obsession. Let it go.

By my early thirties, George continued to make contact with me when he came home to visit his family, but I knew he was doing it either as a habit or obligation. We no longer shared experiences, and instead we became storytellers creating pictures for each other of our life's events.

It didn't help my quest for stability that his mother would announce to me before George had an opportunity to do so of his impending arrival home. There was even a time when George's mom picked up the handset of their phone in her home, dialled my number and handed him the phone after she announced to me first that George was home and wanted to speak with me. I will never forget those moments of silence, visualizing the assumptive image of George grimacing at his mother and reluctantly taking the offered handset.

At this point of our friendship, we were no longer equal participants. I was no longer hearing him. I was not comfortable, and in my discomfort I talked incessantly when we met, without allowing him to contribute to the discussions.

I remember one visit with George in the first home I owned. I think it was the first time he had been in my home, and I was babbling with pride about being a new homeowner. I noticed George periodically checking his watch. It took a few more similar visits, but I started timing those conversations and became very proficient at knowing when the visit was over. It was always exactly an hour. That was his gift to me. That was the sign I needed.

In my mid-thirties, I developed medical symptoms that required surgery, which would take away my dream to have children of my own. During the wait, George had contacted me and wanted a visit. Poor George … I had been wracked with guilt over trying to extend this friendship beyond what was real. I was mad about what was going to be happening to me and upset over my current personal life circumstances.

I had a plan, a plan to say good-bye. A few months before that last visit, I had written a poem about the distance and change in our friendship. I knew I was ready and felt armed for the possible hurt with the poem at hand. I made sure that the visit wasn't in my home, and we agreed to meet at a restaurant. Wouldn't you know it, my sister Nicole picked that day to eat in the same restaurant! Oh well, I had to do this.

We met, did the usual catch up, ate lunch and just minutes before I knew my hour was up, I read my poem to him. I hadn't considered how much this would shock or hurt George. I hadn't taken into account the challenges he was facing in his life. I was doing this for me. That was not me, but it was the me I needed to be in order to move on.

It was about fifteen years after that farewell lunch that I reconnected with my friend. George had kept his promise and hadn't sought me out. The ability to let go took time, but gradually I would go through weeks and months of not wondering how he was or what he was doing. Ivory continued her friendship with George and through her I would hear occasional updates. I assumed he also was receiving updates about me. It wasn't as if we didn't know of our continued journeys, we just didn't seek each other out. Why then, fifteen years later, was it important for me to reach out and renew this friendship? I'm still not sure.

Maybe it was my second opportunity of life after a major surgery that triggered this quest. My matured understanding that love comes in many different forms might have been another reason. Even though I knew how successful George was in his professional role, I wondered how he really was. Maybe I just wanted my friend back. Yes, that was it.

So I gathered courage, after six months of "what ifs," and initiated the first contact. It was hesitant. It was slow on both our parts, but I think we were both pleased to realize that glimpses of a friendship from so long ago were still there.

The safety of online social networks allows you to make contact with a person but also allows the walls and boundaries to remain in place until you reach a level of trust or comfort. George and I started communicating through online writing, and it soon became apparent to me that there was a possibility of renewing this friendship or maybe creating a different one. It felt easy when the words were being typed and wirelessly transferred between us.

The first time we agreed to meet through a videoconference was hard, yet surprisingly normal. The first time we met in person was terrifying, but great. He was still my friend, a little older but still the same. I was honest with George and apologized for letting go of our friendship. I knew I had my friend back and also knew that this renewed friendship, while progressing in a positive manner, was a delicate one.

George is someone I love as a brother, as a friend and unique individual who has had his own battles to overcome. I know he understands and returns those similar feelings. Making those new connections we realized how similar our challenges of life have been and how similar society has viewed our differences from others. His journey of life is as interesting and as different as mine. Maybe someday he will share that journey with others. But since he is so much like me, he would probably prefer to keep things private.

A short while ago, a family member labelled me as having OCD, Obsessive Compulsive Disorder. While I was greatly hurt and highly offended by this unqualified diagnosis, I can understand why this sibling would think this way. I have a tendency to compartmentalize segments of my life and will treat certain aspects with greater focus than others. I do admit to being obsessive, but it is usually only with what I currently love.

This chapter is about my obsession with love, and I could easily include my obsessions of my career or other interests as well. When I became aware of a new educational trend or topic while teaching, I would study and consume everything I could to learn about it. My time put into teaching was sometimes unbalanced and unusually focussed more than it should have been. I also knew that benefits of that time and study were returned through viewing the expressions of my students and parents. This far outweighed my worry of whether teaching was an obsession for me.

My time playing music, making teddy bears and completing other crafts could also be viewed as obsessions, but I tended to view them as a need for self-expression. The feeling of accomplishment and pride in producing something that brings great joy to others was not an obsession for me. It was and continues to be a gift. These passions could be seen as obsessions; instead, I regard them as preferences.

I prefer reading romances for a reason. In addition to having the ability to scare myself silly by reading other genres, I believe in love. I have witnessed and been the recipient of love my entire life: the love I receive from my family and their ongoing faith in me, the love of friends, and the unique relationships I have had the opportunity to encounter, the love of unexpected occurrences when you meet someone of interest. Love is all around me, and I am constantly the recipient of the gestures of love. Whether it is a child's excitement of being with me while learning or a gesture from a family member or friend who tells me they care, I have always been surrounded by love.

Then there is the magic of intimate love between two people that I have not yet experienced. I have had a recurring dream of being with a person. I know it is a dream. I wake up with the feeling of being loved. I know it is a man. I know it is someone who knows me well. I also know that it is a way of helping me heal after I have been hurt in some way. This dream is full of the giving of love to each other and feeling totally trusted and supported. It is a reassurance that someone believes in me and loves me. It settles me and lets me believe in me. Maybe someday ...

The joy of those I love and the possibilities to come

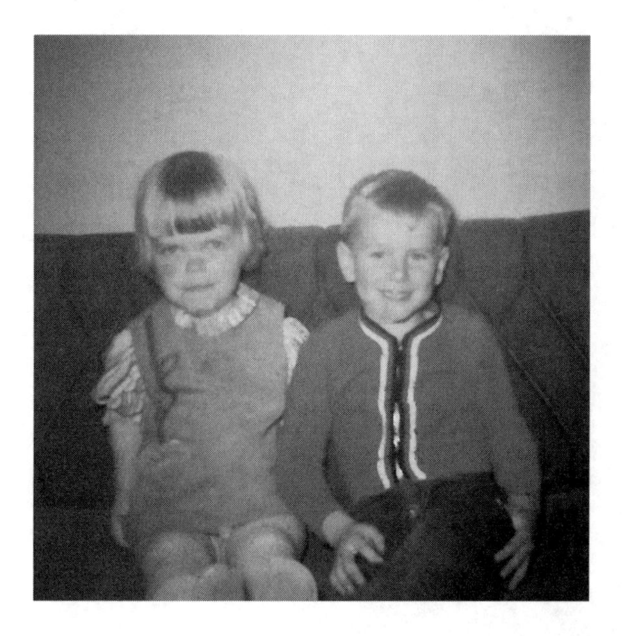

George and me.

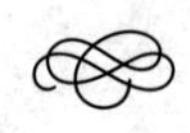

Chapter 8

The pain of a kiss, of a dance or a hug, these things
I cannot miss since I've never known them

Many years ago, Dad said to me, "Why don't you just be a secretary?" It was at some point in my career as a teacher when I was struggling with a professional challenge, and my entire life seemed to be consumed with this problem of which I now have no recollection.

My dad was a very observant individual, and I assume he was seeing me as missing out on many aspects of life while I strived to be so "normal." I was raised to be independent. I was raised with the belief that nothing can stop me. My parents instilled in me the expectation that I would be educated, I would have a job and I would give back to others. I worked hard to excel in those areas. It took me a long time to realize how much time and energy it would take for me to portray success at being "normal." He was so right in making this comment. Unfortunately, I didn't hear what he was actually saying.

My dad was not saying that to fill the role of a secretary was of lesser value or accomplishment. Dad was saying that he was worried about me, and he wanted more than what I thought was normal. Normal for me was measurement of my success in my career, my relationships with family and friends and my independence. But I also felt that I was failing in one important aspect of life: personal relationships. I cannot recall any conversations with my parents, siblings or friends about creating intimate relationships with others or my lack of achievement in being a sexual being. The topics of dating, sex and personal preferences in relationships were never discussed.

Being physically close to others is foreign for me. I have been the recipient of many hugs, but do not seem to offer the same number back to others. Catching another person with an arm and gathering them in for a hug, chest to chest, is a challenge, especially when I am standing there and feeling the need to give or receive a hug. My siblings and their children have mastered the art of hugging, and we seem to now reflect other families who commonly hug in greeting or departure. But for me it remains an uncertainty. I wrote a poem long ago with the words, "How do you make up for the feet?" It was in reference to my hesitation of wanting to give a hug to another, but knowing that unless I reached out and hugged that person's hips or waist, there was going to be that moment of uncomfortable hesitancy.

My comfort in reaching out to someone is better when we are physical equals. If that person is a child, my inclination to offer a hug increases. If an adult is sitting or my height is equal to them, I will reach out. I have had to work hard to ignore my natural resistance in initiating a hug with someone standing. Most adults of similar height quickly reach out, grab a shoulder, and offer a hug before that person has time to choose. The gesture I make of opening my arms and waiting for that person to bend down, so that I am hugging their shoulders and not their waist, remains a very uncomfortable moment for me. There is a chance that the invitation to hug will be denied, and I am left there with my arms wide open. It has happened. There has been more than one person who has repelled my gesture and instead offered me a hand to shake.

By the time I reached my teenage years the concept of flirting, dating and connecting to someone special was an expected norm that I assumed I would be part of. I started attending school dances along with my peers and loved watching others on the dance floor, but I never danced. Years ago, it was not common as it is today for a group of young people of either gender to just gather on the dance floor and dance. My generation had strict rules of dancing, including the idea that it only involved a couple of a mixed gender; teenagers of today just dance.

I didn't quit attending school dances even when I was a repeated wallflower sitting at a table watching the dancing throughout the evening. As a young adult, wedding receptions were another time when I would stay and watch those dancing. After each dance, I would go home and dance by myself, mirroring the steps I had observed. The connection between people while dancing was a dialogue of words through body motions, and I loved observing that type of communicating. No one ever questioned why I wasn't dancing. No one came forward and asked me to dance. Well … one did.

My high school friends and I, once the majority of us had reached legal drinking age, started frequenting a bar across the river. It was a large building at the corner entrance of the town that housed many different businesses in the past, including various restaurants and bars. The theme of the bar at the time was country, and the band playing was sticking to the common line dancing and two-step songs of that era. It was one of the rare nights when the group I was with were all females. Most of my friends were getting up to dance with other patrons of the bar, and I was in my common position watching from the table.

About an hour into watching others dance, a tall male approached our table, came closer to me, and asked if I wanted to dance. Being young and totally reliant on gearing my responses based on my friend's expressions, I looked around the table and noted their reactions. Their faces were reflecting disbelief and horror. Why? Someone just asked me to dance. What was so wrong with that?

Being the person others wanted me to be, I knew what I had to say. I thanked the man, but said I didn't dance. That was the first time but not the last time I would say that lie. Immediately afterwards, my group of friends decided they needed to leave. Their embarrassment at the situation was short lived. Mine was not.

I have danced throughout my lifetime, but just not in the formal sense in the presence of other adults dancing. It started after my university years when I was trying to lose weight and discovered a series of Jane Fonda aerobic dance videos. I loved learning the basic dance steps knowing that this movement was also helping my goal of better health. Once teaching, I made sure that dance was part of any music program I was responsible for, and would eagerly encourage young, hesitant students to get up and dance with the rest of us.

Still though, I did not dance at formal adult dances even though my soul was crying for me to get out there and move. Dancing is letting go and allowing your emotions to express themselves through movement. I know that today I would be welcomed with other single dancers who think nothing of hopping onto the dance floor and moving their feet to the rhythm of the music. But like other things I only do in private, the years of holding back and hiding the truth of who I am or want to be have created an emotional barrier between me and the me people expect me to be.

My lack of intimacy with someone special took years for me to understand and accept. My fears, my anxieties and my need for controls influenced my lack of opportunities and moments. Back when I said "I cannot miss them since I have never known them" it was false. I do miss them even when I have never known them. Reading about or watching fictitious sexual acts between couples is not reality, but it can be informative. Observing couples interact in front of me is no longer hurtful to see, but instead is a celebration of the way life should be. Today, I proudly say if questioned that I am asexual. Am I, though?

I could add many more items to that list I started thirty years ago of what I am not, or what I have not yet experienced. I was never a skier or a swimmer but loved to be near water. I seem to be top heavy and repeated swimming lessons only confirmed my belief that my head weighed more than the rest of my body. The only cars I have driven were my own, and I have never test driven a car before purchasing one. I have never experienced the thrill of racing around by myself on a quad, a motorcycle or a snowmobile. I have never been on a date or been involved intimately with another person. I was never a mother to my own children but have loved others.

Even though I believed the dire prediction of long ago of my expected demise, I yearned for what others were accomplishing in their adult lives. When you are raised with the assumption that you will be married and have children one day then it is tough to consider other choices in life even when the opportunities or possibilities seem to be disappearing. I was strong in my belief that in order to find a life mate you had to let nature take its course and provide those opportunities. The opportunity to find a life mate was hampered by my unwillingness to let go of past beliefs and feelings. During one of my counselling sessions early in my teaching career, when I was talking about my continued single status, this counsellor suggested I try to find that special someone through online dating. At that time, sites that encouraged you to post your picture and name online were just emerging. The idea of me doing something like that was beyond me.

I thought having children wasn't possible for many reasons, yet for a long time I had a strong urge to be a mother. I had been acting like a mother already, caring for others, doing for others, and that idea of having a special someone that I would care for was a dream and hope. I would hold my friends' babies, my nieces and nephews, and dream of that someday. I truly believed that someday would be one day. I even made out plans for adapting a baby's living space so I could physically take care of a baby. I wasn't considering the mechanics involved in producing a child; my dream always started at the beginning of that child's life.

To share with others my dream was futile because I already knew that many would not see this same dream for me. Gradually, I quit holding babies. My nieces and nephews were young toddlers or older by this time. I started to express to others my preference of interacting with children once they were walking or talking when babies were offered for me to hold. My desire to hold and cuddle a baby remained, but I grew tired of others watching me closely, hovering in anticipation of rescuing the infant from me. This someone was usually one who did not know or trust me. It would happen when I would be switching positions with the baby in my arms. The manner of me carefully making this change was different from the norm and that seemed to frighten others. Rarely in a group setting did I hold an infant without someone feeling the need to rescue me, or especially the infant.

I would watch and wait though. Every child grows older and there would always be one day that I would feel okay to interact with that child. This was a special time of fantasy for that child and me. For the child, who most often was less than three years of age, I was a fellow playmate who only wanted to play with them. The child truly had no idea that I was an adult and only wanting to be playing with someone else. I knew this playtime was limited, and eventually the child would look at me as an adult. That awareness usually happened as they started school and then the questions would begin.

I have spent a large part of my adulthood focussed on children and will probably continue to do so for the rest of my life. Children are pure spirits who only want to explore their world. They think without boundaries, without walls, and look to others for answers. I have watched children grow into caring, competent young adults. I have also watched life's challenges interfere with that growth and repeatedly wanted to rescue that child from their current circumstances.

When I reached my early thirties, life was full of busy activities. Between my teaching, my leadership within my professional organization and other obligations, I didn't worry about missing out on my dreams to be married or to be a mother. Women in their forties were having children, and I felt I had a lot of time to find those opportunities. While my heart and head felt there was plenty of time, physically my body had decided my chances of having children were coming to an end.

I had always had difficulty each month during my monthly cycle. The pacing around my parents' house trying to walk off the pain was patterned by the repeated path I took trying not to wake other members of my family while walking throughout the night. In my teenage years, I was admitted to hospital for the pain a few times, and on one of those occasions surgery was performed to remove cysts from my ovaries. Eventually, the proper balance of medicines was prescribed, and I was able to sustain some control of the monthly pain.

By my mid-thirties, changes in my cycle required further investigation. In addition to the endometriosis I had learned to cope with for twenty years, I was now diagnosed as having fibroids. The first specialist I saw didn't feel surgery was needed. Instead, her prescription was that I should get pregnant, but I would need to conceive a child within the next year before the symptoms became worse. After getting over her outrageous message, I laughed for a long time. To me, it was ludicrous that I would purposely have a child in that manner, for that reason.

The second specialist I saw was a little more realistic, and regrettably recommended that I needed to have a hysterectomy. Feeling the need for control, I engineered the date of the surgery for May, so my expected six-week recuperation time would end just as summer holidays were beginning in schools. I do not have a lot of memories of the actual surgery process, but recall waking up to the sound of crying babies.

The hospital had placed me on the maternity ward after my surgery. The second evening after hearing the sounds of crying babies that entire day, a nurse who thought she was doing something appropriate brought to my bedside a newborn baby for me to see. I did not sleep that night. Instead, I wrote.

I had brought an empty journal with me thinking this might be a new journey full of emotions that needed to be recorded, and was so thankful I had it. I somehow climbed down from the bed using the metal handrail as steps and retrieved my journal, a pen and my pain meds. For the rest of the night I wrote. I look back at that particular writing and can see such disbelief and sorrow I had at that time. However, I was still me; I was also forming a plan.

At five the next morning, I found a chair, dragged it over to the pay phone in the hallway and called my parents' home. My mom was an early riser, and I knew she would be close to getting up at that time. I did not say much to her, but only asked her to come and get me. She was a few hours away but by noon was present to take me home. During that time, I had convinced the doctor and staff that I was well enough to recuperate in my parents' home.

There have been times in my life that being different, or being little, has been an advantage, especially during an argument, and this was one of those times. My story of persuasion involved comparing the high beds and items in the hospital, including the height of the toilet seat, to what my parents could offer me at home. It was convincing. Looking back now, I totally disregarded the amount of stress this may have put on my parents to care for me for the next few weeks. I just wanted to flee and get away from the sound of crying babies.

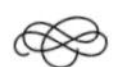

I feel I may not have explored all the intricacies of being intimate with others. However, I have never stopped exploring and will keep exploring all the possibilities of my life. I have visions of where I should be, or what I should be doing. Most of these visions happened while sleeping, and usually took place just before I was to wake up in the morning. It took me a long time to pay attention to these visions and realize that my subconscious feelings were making themselves known. During my formal teaching years, these visions helped create solutions to challenges at school. These visions have warned me when I was travelling a path or journey that was not in my best interest. There were many mornings when I would eagerly share my latest educational vision of change with my administrators. These visions have also shown me possibilities I should pay attention to.

One of the most important of my life saw me living with my mother, or rather seeing my mother living in my home with me. Mom's drive to create normalcy for me while growing up was something I had never forgotten, but I had no idea how I could reciprocate. Mom was a very independent person, and it was difficult for her to accept the assistance of others. An amusing story relates to the routine followed when Mom and Dad would go away for a vacation. The teenagers of the family would take over the cooking chores at home until we knew the expected time of Mom's return. We then would work at making sure everything was in its place, with the counters and stovetop scrubbed clean. We would then wait for Mom to arrive home and watch for the first thing she would do after greeting us. Most often, she would enter the kitchen, go to the sink, wet the dish cloth and wipe down the already cleaned counter and stovetop. The kids would then all smile and nod in agreement that Mom was home and she was once again taking over her kitchen.

After my hysterectomy surgery in the mid-1990s, I started questioning whether teaching was something I wanted to do for the rest of my career. If not, what did I want to do? One of my dream jobs was to become a travel consultant. In my fourteenth year of teaching, I decided to complete a correspondence course in travel, and started to volunteer at a local travel agency Saturday mornings. By the end of that year, I had finished all book and computer studies, and was preparing to write my exam to be a certified Level 1 Travel Consultant. It was at this time that the manager of the agency I was volunteering for offered me a temporary position that would last for a half a year, until a fellow consultant returned from maternity leave. This was a great opportunity for me. I was questioning so many things in my life after the surgery and to have this door of change open was such a positive moment.

The request for a half-year's leave was granted by my school board, and I eagerly started work early in July without even considering the need for a summer vacation. The opportunity to greet a variety of people and the challenge of meeting their travel needs was just what I needed at this time. There were many similarities in what I was doing working in sales as compared to teaching. I started regarding airline seat sales as report card times. The amount of hours selling and completing ticket work during an airline promotion reminded me of the frantic times teachers go through trying to teach while completing those required term reports. The biggest surprise was the discrepancy in pay. I would joke to others that what I would pay in taxes as a teacher was equivalent to what my income was as a travel consultant.

As the months went on, I started missing the consistencies and order of teaching and looked forward to returning to my first career. For most teachers, there is comfort in knowing daily which students will be walking through your door and what your schedule will look like. Working in travel sales, every day was very unpredictable in terms of whom you would see and the duties to complete. I even found myself at times wanting to put some of the more trying travel customers into a time out.

I had the opportunity to participate in two familiarization trips during this placement at the travel agency, and planned a third trip at my own expense. I had been promising my niece, Yvette, a trip for a long while and since she was newly married, I thought I better schedule a trip soon prior to this young couple starting their family. We arranged to travel to Mexico and soon afterwards, Mom decided she would come along as well. I was so glad Yvette was with me for this trip. I had travelled alone other times with Mom, but really had no inkling of what was progressing or regressing within her mind until that trip took place.

Many of us began to see changes in Mom's personality long before she was diagnosed with vascular dementia. During this trip, Mom was okay during times when we were relaxing on the beach or viewing the shops. The week was full of relaxation and sun. I did learn the negative effects of drinking too many margaritas the night before travelling on a double decker bus to the Mayan ruins, but for the most part, it was a memorable trip.

There were unexpected moments, though, that gave both Yvette and I some challenges. Crowded, noisy, unexpected times would shut Mom down to a point where she would put her hands to her head and refuse to communicate with us. The first time it happened was as we landed at the airport in Mexico.

The worst time happened while we were taking a rather noisy dinner cruise along the coast, and she insisted she wanted to get off the boat immediately.

Yvette and I attempted to share our concerns with family members after we returned, but most just excused Mom's actions as part of her age and personality. Gradually, though, other members of our family noticed other changes in Mom such as her withdrawal from various organizations she had long been a part of, and her tendency to prepare prepackaged frozen food for most of the meals. We did not realize it at the time, but Dad was compensating considerably for Mom's failing cognitive abilities. It was only after the passing of my father that family members agreed that Mom's memory issues were significant. It was only after his death that Mom was willing to discuss her own health issues.

After Dad's passing, many of the siblings living near Mom would make a greater effort to provide various supports that Dad had probably been providing for Mom for many years. One of my roles, in addition to being her social coordinator, was to help Mom live independently during the summer months at our cabin at the lake. Mom's favourite place was the cabin, but her time there was becoming too much of a change for her. For a few summers, the two of us would spend many months at the lake. I would commute for the final month of the school year with Mom being fairly safe on her own during the day. Other family members would join us, but for the most part, it would just be Mom and me.

The progression of Mom's dementia became even more noticeable. It was at the cabin during one of those summers that

I asked Mom whether she would be interested in moving into my home. I had discussed the idea with many of my siblings ahead of time and most supported the idea. My sister Allison, the one who worked in home care, was the only one who felt that this idea might not be the best one for me.

In many ways, Allison was right, but it took some time for those reasons to become apparent. In the fall of that same school year, I moved all my personal items and set up my living space in the basement area. Mom's possessions were moved into the upstairs portion of my house. I had recently been transferred to a new school closer to my home, so I was able to be home for most midday meals. Mom continued to drive for that first year, and while she didn't travel too far from our community, she would often continue to take other ladies out shopping, etc.

During that first year, Mom was able to contribute to many daily tasks including heating meals for lunch, washing the dishes, completing the laundry and assisting with the grocery shopping. Her reading and hand-sewing abilities were two skills that seemed to last longer than many other activities. Most days, she filled her time reading books or the newspaper and working on a particular quilt.

Gradually, however, I started noticing how much Mom was becoming more reliant on me. Her ability to make simple meals or contribute to other daily chores lessened and eventually ceased. I had to make sure every appliance she was still using had an automatic shutoff, and I encouraged her not to use the stove. Mom eventually stopped driving, which to many of us was a huge relief. Little accidents such as spills or stains found in the carpet were becoming more common. I also began ensuring clean clothes were worn each day by stealing the soiled ones from the bottom of Mom's bed each night.

Mom continued to work hard at masking her diminishing abilities from others, but this was becoming impossible. While she could continue to converse with fluency, at times her understanding of what people were saying to her was a challenge. People would direct a question to Mom, and she often would look to others or me for the answer. Mom found being in crowds daunting and gradually her interest in participating in social groups, even when one of us accompanied her, ended.

From an early age, I had always played the role of mother, and while I did not have the opportunity of having my own children, I did have many experiences of being a parent while my mother was living with me. The difference was those special years were in a sped-up, reverse order to what most parents experience. As days progressed, my duties accumulated, and I found myself worrying more about Mom's safety while I was working. Mike and Nicole were already providing daily support by scheduling times to check up on Mom while I was teaching, but the toll of this support was starting to drain all of us.

It was obvious that the level of care Mom required was more than what my siblings or I could offer. It took months of assessments from Home Care to designate Mom's condition as being severe enough for extended care. The first few scheduled home assessments Mom knew of ahead of time, and she worked hard at putting on a believable show to convince the assessor of her abilities. The third assessment was a planned unexpected one. I suggested the assessor approach the large framed picture of our family members that hung in her living space and ask Mom to identify her children. By this time, Mom's visual recognition and ability to name all seven children and six grandchildren was a challenge for her. Sure enough, when she was unable to name two of her seven children, she decided to inform the assessor instead that those people did not belong in her family.

I have never given birth to a child, never comforted a sick child through all hours of the night, never worried about a teenaged child hoping he or she will arrive home safe. I have, however, experienced a similar feeling of the loss of a child the day Mom was placed into care. I had taken care of Mom, for those few years up to the day she left my home, as if she was my own child. I was the parent in this relationship, and I had always wanted to repay my parents for their years of support. However, I never again wanted to experience the excruciating guilt and loss I experienced the day Mom started receiving care from qualified professionals in a different home.

Mom's continued journey with dementia while in care consisted of many different rides that none of us expected. When I voiced so long ago that I had never experienced a kiss, a dance and a hug and therefore would never miss them, I did not have the maturity or experience of taking a journey such as the one with my mother. During Mom's final years, there were many opportunities to dance, kiss and hug with this person who brought me and my siblings into this world. I will always cherish the opportunities I was fortunate to experience while my mom lived with me and during her final years in care.

Poignant to those memories is the final opportunity we were gifted with from Mom. My mother was physically strong. There were moments during her last months of living when the three siblings living closest to Mom would be called in the middle of the night because of the care facility's certainty that she was about to pass away. Mom was determined, though, and by each morning would rally and be sitting up when we returned to visit after our night of sleepless vigil. At this same time, a reawakened awareness occurred within Mom, and she would comment on topics and relationships with others she had forgotten for years.

It was during one of these opportunities of clarity that I asked Mom if she wanted to talk to each of her children. Her response was, "We could do that." Just hearing that response was a surprise to what she usually could voice. I like to believe she knew what was coming and was using all of her energy to reach out to us a final time.

For some of my siblings, there were increased visits and contacts. For those farther away, I found a common time to call them on my mobile phone and Mom had an opportunity to talk with most of her children on speaker phone. More importantly, my sisters and brothers had been granted an opportunity to speak to her.

Mom passed peacefully in the middle of the night with me quietly beside her. She was my family, my friend and my love. Many have said to me that I lost a period of my life while I focussed my attention on this journey with Mom. Instead, I feel she gave me back life. Our funny, joyous moments together will be cherished for my lifetime. The line of the poem says, "these things I cannot miss since I have never known them." I have known in a different way what being close to someone is, and I still miss those intimate connections.

As friends and family members have moved or passed on, there has been a time for each adjustment and an understanding of how their absence will be changing my life. My expectation is I will find new close connections with others, and I understand that those connections may be different from what others are used to.

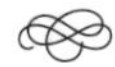

My experiences in my life are not missing; they are just different. I have had unique experiences because of who I am. Doors have been opened and crowded lines have vanished because of the attention I can gather. I have been a part of two commercials on TV that were aired simultaneously to viewers in the province. I represented our local teachers at the provincial level for over twenty years, including those complex times when the provincial bargaining process had broken down. I have represented my profession as a director on our Teachers' Pension Board, and instigated change to governance when I felt it was needed. I have had the opportunity to play music in concerts and at church events. I have been a teacher, a travel agent, and now I am a small home business owner. I am a creator who writes songs and poetry, forms videos of the past and makes teddy bears that bring joy to others. I hope that I will also be able to say soon that I am also one who has written a book. I will continue to absorb life and find those experiences that are fitting for me.

Celebrating special moments in life is important, and for me the year I transitioned from the end of one career to the beginning of another was well timed. It was the year after Mom had passed and my last year as an employed teacher. That memorable calendar year was filled with repeated celebrations and acknowledgements including hosting my own dinner party for more than a hundred and fifty guests.

To me, that special evening was equivalent to any other person's wedding celebration or baby shower. I spent months planning and organizing the dinner, making sure those who had influenced my teaching years were included on the guest list. Every detail, including the decorations on the tables and the colour theme of the event, was planned out. The evening passed quickly, and for me was filled with abundant attention and love.

During that evening, two touching memories stand out for me. For a person who prefers to be in control of her environment, I was high from the bubbles of excessive planning and decision-making. I had asked my youngest niece, Abigail, to provide entertainment and informed her of the exact song I wanted her to sing. Abby is a wonderful adult who has always exhibited great independence. She brought tears to my eyes when she performed a song of her own choosing that was a much better choice.

The second wonderful surprise was when I had concluded my words of thanks to the guests and announced that it was time to serve the cake. My grandnieces, including Adriana, grabbed my hands as I passed their table and eagerly joined me at the table where the cakes were ready to be served. The picture of them with me at that moment was priceless.

That year of celebration also was unique because of the six planned vacations celebrating family and friends. The first, with

Ivory, was a quick trip to England to visit our niece Abby who was working at that time as a substitute teacher in London. The next month, I met Allison and her husband in San Diego, spending time watching the ocean waves and renewing our "sister" relationship after Mom's passing. The celebration of the marriage of Greg's son, Neil, granted an opportunity for three of the four sisters to have a weekend trip to the coast of British Columbia where we completed the third trip.

In celebration of my retirement from teaching and the commencement of Abby acquiring her first teaching position, a trip to see the Toronto Blue Jays baseball team play in California was quickly added to the year of celebration in early summer. A trip to Calgary to connect with my LP friends at a weekend conference and to spend time with some of my relatives on Mom's side concluded the summer. The final trip of the year was planned later in the fall, and it seemed fitting to be part of the year's theme of reflection and change. Ivory and I travelled to visit our close friend George, from whom I had felt at one point so long ago that distance was needed. It was a wonderful time getting to know more about George's life and the city he resided in.

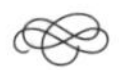

I have always wanted to create a sensory room for average-height people to experience what Little People encounter every day. I think if a stranger or even a misguided friend lived in my environment for a brief time, their understanding and regard for those who are different would change. My dream would include a large room with the furniture and fixtures placed in proportion to what I experience. Instead of a doorknob and lock at waist height, they would be above the shoulders for that average person. Light switches and doorbells would be way above their heads and out of reach. They would have to jump up onto chair seats that are set above their waist and balance on wobbly stools or turned-over garbage cans to reach items within cupboards. They would be invited to experience extreme balancing acts such as carrying boiling pots of water up and down step stools whose steps are as high as your knees. Just the repeated simple action of climbing up and down stairs with the height of the stair adjusted in proportion to that with which most Little People contend would be an excellent simulation of the energy needed to live our daily lives. But these people, who without thought or empathy, tell me how tragic it is to be who I am and express sympathy to me because I was never married or had children, will never experience that type of life I have encountered.

I am now riding a bike once again because of what I saw while sleeping. I saw myself riding a two-wheeler. As a child, I rode a bicycle with training wheels but never gained the full independence of riding a two-wheeler because of my inability to touch the ground from the seat. I had seen other Little People on bikes and knew riding was possible. However, as you become an adult and are busy with commitments, those dreams and wishes that you once had do not seem as important.

Learning to ride a bike in your mid-fifties to some could be seen as dangerous or immature. For me, I knew that if I was able to ride a bike I would have another means of mobility as walking becomes a greater challenge as I age. I was right. It took me a few months to learn how to ride the custom bike I had purchased, but biking is a godsend for me. It still is a scary thing moving at a speed faster than walking without any supports, but it is a new freedom. It also reminded me that it is okay to fall. I felt free when I took my first independent spill, got up and kept going.

It's okay to fall, it's okay to go down paths where you shouldn't be, but it's not okay to quit trying. There will always be a need to seek new avenues and new journeys that I should explore. Some of these experiences will take me on a different path in my life. Some of these experiences will provide a new lesson to learn. I will treasure all of them.

The gift of a kiss, of a dance, of a hug, these things and more I can experience

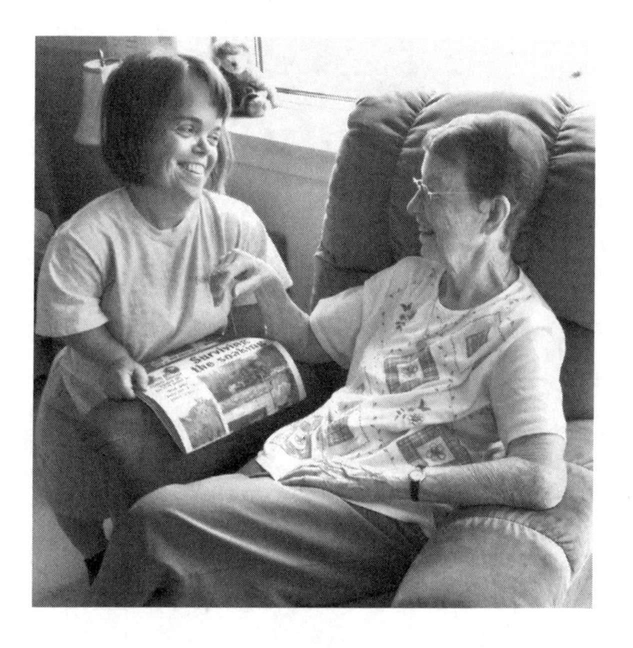

My brother Greg captured this photo of Mom and me.

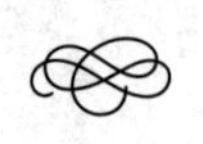

Chapter 9

The question of being normal will never be forgotten

So what is 'normal'? The question of being normal is based on the answers related to how we perceive the world around us. The definition of normal would be based on a strict set of rules we acquire through observation and the limited experiences of youth. To say that question will never be forgotten implies the importance of wanting to be normal.

As a teenager and young adult wanting to be the same, needing to belong, it was understandable that I would see myself as different. It was understandable that during that particular period others would view me as so different. I had worked so hard and succeeded in masking my differences, but continued to question how normal I was.

My family was as normal or as average as any other family. We were lucky and are still so fortunate for what we have. While other families close to us were coping with grave hardships and loss, we seemed to be fortunate in our health and lucky in surviving any accidents. The family I assumed I would one day have of my own has not been achieved, but that is only if you adhere to one specific definition of the word "family." My family is kin. My family is friends. My family is even, at times, strangers.

My friends were, and are, those to whom I am close. The innocent, immature view of having that one confidante who shared everything was long ago my view of what I thought as normal. Society today has given us mixed perceptions of who our friends are by means of access to social networking. My perception of friendship has changed. It is based on values gained from shared experiences, understandings and trust. I have been fortunate in my opportunities to be engaged with a variety of individuals. I feel lucky to have known the ones whom I no longer am in contact with and love the opportunities I have in getting to know new friends.

The reaction of strangers seeing someone as different as me is also normal and will continue to be a part of my life. I may become tired and impatient with their responses and rude actions, but that too is also normal. To hope that everyone I encounter is comfortable enough in their own presence to allow differences in others is a wish or a dream, not a reality.

While the question of being 'normal' was part of the poem I had written so many years ago, for the majority of my life, I did not pay attention to what was or was not normal. It was only when I was experiencing unexplained medical symptoms that my 'normal' was forever altered.

The prediction so long ago that had me believing that my

life would only be half of what others could expect was becoming a brighter beacon as I was approaching my forties. That image of a flashing light indicating how much time was left had increased in intensity and speed. At the same time, unknown physical symptoms were making themselves known, and for a thirty-something-year-old they were not common.

Each year, particularly in the winter months, I would have extreme pain in one joint in my body, but the location of the pain would change from year to year. Varieties of diagnoses were shared after each investigation and possible surgical interventions recommended.

As the arrival of my fortieth year loomed closer, I started to panic. My eyesight was changing and at times I would temporarily lose focus in my vision. My ability to hold and grasp objects without dropping them weakened. My arms and the back of my head would lose sensation at unpredictable times. Most noticeable seemed to be my ability to walk. I was experiencing unusual leg numbness and pain that restricted my steps. At times, I struggled to move, having to concentrate in order to force my legs to move one step at a time.

The physical challenges were beyond my understanding, and I was beginning to believe that what those doctors had said to me as an adolescent was becoming true. A part of me, though, the part that had always walked into battles willing to fight, wanted more: more understandings, more explanations and more time.

The change of my eyesight was diagnosed as cataracts. The fast rate and intensity of the cataract growth resulted in being seen by a top specialist in the province as an emergency patient. Professionals felt that whatever was causing other symptoms in my body was also influencing my eyesight. The eye surgeries occurred within a month of each other. The first surgery was a learning experience for the hospital medical staff after they had to rescue me from the floor at the entrance of the hospital while I was leaving.

After the second eye surgery, the professionals learned another lesson about Little People. In addition to making sure a smaller body is well hydrated during surgery, they also found out, after the fact, that the span in holding a book is less distance for a person with shorter arms. I had never acquired the ability to focus both of my eyes at the same time. Interpreting 3-D pictures and movies had always been a challenge for me. Knowing that, the specialist recommended that my replacement lenses be two different focal lengths, one eye for long distance and one eye for reading distance. Unfortunately, the doctor doing the assessment forgot about my short arms and made my second eye lens for someone with longer arms. I can successfully read without correction if I place reading material about a foot farther than my reach.

In January of 2000, I completed an Internet search for the current location of the doctor who, so many years ago, was of great support for my parents. This specialist now resided in British Columbia, working in a genetics clinic. I contacted her by telephone and her sympathetic response to my numerous questions was well received. She realized I was lacking in the latest medical knowledge of achondroplasia and needed to seek counsel from a local genetic doctor. She provided a name, and I was successful in getting a referral to this specialist in our province. However, I would have to wait.

Referrals to specialists always take time and by then, I did not question the half-year wait required. At this point, I was struggling with left hip and right shoulder pain. The doctor quickly decided a full body Magnetic Resonance Imaging, MRI, and referral to a neurologist was necessary. That was the first of many instances when I would be placed on an emergency status and would not have to wait as long for my next medical appointment or tests.

At this same genetic appointment, I also asked the specialist about the longevity prediction that had been shared with me so long ago. There was disbelief in the doctor's eyes and anger in his expression. He quickly reassured me that the information I had been given was false, and that those with skeletal dysplasia, especially dwarves with achondroplasia, live long lives comparable to an average person.

There was no time for blame because within a month's time from that appointment I had my first appointment with a neurologist. This also initiated a new pattern of challenges for me. The hospital was a teaching hospital, and rarely did I see the specialist before a student resident had reviewed my case and completed an examination. As a child, I did not question this. It was very frustrating as an adult seeking the best advice and diagnosis.

This first neurologist was an ethical one and clearly admitted he had limited knowledge of the neurological complications of a dwarf. Within a few months, I was headed back to this teaching hospital for my first MRI. If you have a fear of enclosed spaces or any unfortunate memories related to the medical world, undergoing an MRI is one of your greatest challenges. In addition to my general anxiety of medical interventions and having to enter a hospital for this test, I was also required to lie still without moving for ninety minutes in a long tube. MRIs have since advanced and the time needed to capture images has since been greatly reduced.

The first time was long and exhausting. I have had seventeen additional MRIs since then, and have become quite comfortable at entering the tube and waiting out the necessary time span. I have also become very knowledgeable and proactive in what pillow supports, positions and music I prefer hearing during these examinations.

The results of a MRI back then were foreign to me, and it took some time to learn to interpret the results. By the second appointment in March of 2001, the true understanding of my condition became clear. My appointment was with an orthopaedic surgeon, who would be the first of many surgeons I would meet in the next five years. I went alone to the appointment confident I would be okay. I was not.

While I did not hear everything, by this time I was recording all medical conversations into a journal, which came in handy after this memorable appointment. The surgeon began by explaining the basics of what a MRI captures, particularly the images within my spine. Words such as atrophy, signal intensity, compression and damage were becoming part of my awareness. All my current symptoms could be explained by his diagnosis, the gravity of which was finally reaching me. What I heard for the first time and would hear for many years afterwards, was that I had a condition of spinal stenosis and the severity of the condition ranged from moderate to severe depending on the position within the spine.

This doctor's gloomy prediction was focussed on a distinct area of my spine just below my skull. He indicated that signals leading from my brain to my spine were being interrupted by the compression of the cord caused by the undersized opening of my skull (called the foramen magnum) and the space within my spinal column. He went on to say he could see that the cord was already starting to show permanent damage or atrophy where it had been in distress for many years. This doctor also calmly explained that my life expectancy would depend on whether surgery was possible. The last thing he said to me was that I needed to protect myself from any falls or jarring of the spine because such an occurrence would lead to instant death.

What I did between this appointment and driving back home is blank. I remember thinking while I was driving that I should not be driving. I went home and started a new research window on my computer that remained open for some time after that. I became an "obsessive" expert on this spinal condition. A few days after that appointment, I searched and found online the name of a hospital that specialized in surgeries for patients with skeletal dysplasia. The likelihood of receiving support from a facility out of the country and so far away seemed to be beyond me. Little did I know that possibility of support would come true.

Succinctly, I needed surgery to relieve the pressure on my spinal cord in order to live, and it would not be an easy journey to achieve. Visualize this journey as a series of mini-wars with many battles between: the wars that took place between me and my specialists; the wars with those who assured me they "thought" they knew how to do this unknown procedure, and me assuring them I had no interest in being their first test case; the wars with those who would take me on as a patient and then leave the province, requiring a restart to the referral process once again; the wars with those who would leave my file closed on their desks without addressing their promised outcomes for many months; and my favourite, the wars that happened between my specialists, who would unknowingly recommend each other as the better person to complete the surgery.

At the same time, there was the battle of continuing my existence. I was working in a teaching position where young students, having behavioural or emotional problems, came to a special program in our school division. Students would physically hit out at others, including their teachers, and now I was cognizant of the risk and ramifications of being hit. My focus was finding ways to prevent being hit because the guilt of that person doing the hitting would forever affect their life if something disastrous happened.

Meanwhile, I was in another battle: to maintain the energy and focus to do my professional job as best as I could. Eventually, I had to recognize that I could not and had to accept the consideration of part-time prolonged sick leaves. Having to admit that I was not able to complete my full job was an emotional struggle that lasted until my eventual retirement some ten years later.

In the spring of 2004, Dad passed away and as I was saying my last words to him, I promised him that I would keep on living. Not only would I live, I would celebrate living. I had seen the toll this medical war had taken on my parents for the past four years and wanted to reassure him that I would keep fighting to live.

That same year, in the summer, I decided to attend my first

Little People of America conference. It was time to seek advice from those who actually knew what being a dwarf meant. The annual LPA National conferences were held in different US cities each July. That year, it was being held in San Francisco. Ivory and I travelled together, looking forward to exploring a city of interest. While I was intrigued to be attending my first conference and, more importantly, attending the scheduled medical consultations I had prearranged, my focus was not on the social or interactive opportunities that most Little People and their families enjoyed while attending.

For my entire life, I have bravely walked into new settings and situations knowing what I must do to make others comfortable. My first time attending a LPA conference took me to the other perspective of what people see when I approach them. Ivory and I arrived at the conference hotel, checked in and decided that I should register for the conference before we planned any other activities. While checking in, I had noticed a few other Little People nearby but was not particularly concerned. I didn't realize that the comfort of having Ivory with me was the key.

Ivory peeled off towards the gift shop as we were walking towards the conference registration area. All of a sudden, I was alone amongst a huge number of adults who were just like me. They walked, they talked and they were fully functioning humans, and I could not help but stare.

The majority of these national conferences have over two thousand participants each year. Not only was I immediately overwhelmed with the visual picture I was seeing, I was also panicking because the vast repetition of images that for me should have been normal were so foreign. Outside, I maintained a façade of a calm adult; inside I had reverted to all those emotions of fear and anxiety that I had experienced as a child. I wanted to hide.

Ivory soon found me, and I remember telling her to never leave me alone again for the rest of the conference. She ignored that request, as she knew I was only having a brief meltdown for that moment. The funny thing is that Ivory then, or other family members at future conferences, never had any moments of discomfort being amongst a room full of Little People. Ivory and other members of my family have lived their lives with a dwarf, and seeing other Little People did not faze them.

By the end of the conference, I had made connections with a variety of individuals and to my surprise, many of them admitted the same initial moments of discomfort at being amongst a group of Little People. How we perceive ourselves on a daily basis is entirely different from how others perceive us.

Eventually, my eyes became used to what I was seeing, and I started looking beyond my first impression. The opportunity to share and trade practicalities of adapting to live in an average person's world was wonderful. One of the best sessions I attended during this first conference was an informal gathering of female Little People talking about general issues and intimate concerns, something I had never done before.

I came to realize the many positive benefits of interactions at LPA conferences. In addition to the learning opportunities and access to provided supports, we as LPs were allowed to let go of our expected images and just be ourselves. Some seemed to let go a little bit beyond my expectations. There was no one you had to educate, there was no one you had to comfort and there was no one you had to perform for. It was also the opportunity and setting to perhaps find a life partner.

The scheduled medical appointments for LPA conference attendees were offered free, with medical specialists from all over the continent attending these annual events and volunteering their time. This LPA Medical Advisory Board was, and still is, the lifeline of this organization. With over two hundred distinct types of dwarfism and their individual medical needs, the access the LPA offers to parents and individuals with dwarfism is exceptional. During the week I attended, I was scheduled for three appointments with specialists.

The first LP specialist was a geneticist who once again confirmed my chances for longevity and provided advice on how to sustain life as a middle-aged LP. The second visit was with an orthopaedic surgeon who was a Little Person as well. He eventually would become one of the surgeons involved in the surgery I would have the following year. It was at the third appointment with a renowned neurosurgeon, very well respected in the Little People community, that I gained the most attention.

After briefly meeting the neurosurgeon, he asked if he could call in some of his associates and soon the hotel room they were using for consultations was filled with various professionals. The first question I was asked after a second neurological examination was performed was, "What are you doing still alive?" Well, that was something to think about in so many ways.

The condition I had at the top of my spine was very rare in people with achondroplasia and extremely rare in dwarf adults my age. Usually this condition was diagnosed when you were a child and if the diagnosis was missed or surgery was not provided, the likelihood of reaching adult age was not possible.

For the first time since starting this medical journey, I felt I was making progress. The specialists conferred and agreed that, while they themselves were collectively highly experienced in performing surgeries on LPs, there was only one surgeon they knew of that would have the ability to attempt this surgery. This surgeon worked alongside the orthopaedic surgeon from my second conference appointment at Johns Hopkins Medicine (JHM)[10] in Baltimore, Maryland. It was, coincidentally, the same medical facility that I had researched four years before this conference.

Johns Hopkins Medicine, specifically Johns Hopkins Hospital, is not one building. It is a city of buildings within the city of Baltimore, Maryland. Over twenty large buildings are a part of the hospital. Each common department of a hospital seems to be its own building. Over forty thousand people work at JHM. What had grabbed my interest four years previously was the department titled Greenburg Center for Skeletal Dysplasia,[11] an entire department devoted to the medical wellness of Little People.

It would take another ten months before I would succeed in achieving the surgery at Johns Hopkins as an international patient. My body during this time was fading, and my energy to continue the battle was becoming nonexistent. Four months before the necessary surgery, I lost the ability to drive my car because my condition was affecting my arm strength. Three months before my surgery I received notice from the provincial medical authorities denying my request for surgery out of province. I almost gave up fighting this battle. The province gave as its reason for denial that a specialist in Canada would certainly be qualified to complete this surgery. They just didn't know who or where.

My family was not willing to let go. We now knew that there was a possibility of a positive outcome. We just didn't know what precedents would be involved in creating that outcome. The battle with the province in seeking medical financial permission for a referral and eventual surgery outside of Canada was impressive. My sister Nicole, along with other family members and friends, became part of my army. First, Nicole contacted various suggested specialists in Canada and confirmed to the provincial authorities that there was no one in our nation qualified or willing to take on this challenge. At one point, the battle became a political one with the local Members of the Legislative Assembly prepared to present my case to the provincial authorities.

Within weeks after a different neurologist in the province took on the battle, the war with ministry officials was won, and I was granted permission to receive medical help outside of Canada. Soon after that, I started my travels with financial assistance for most travel expenses provided by a charity that is well known within our province for their annual telethons.

A series of pre-surgical examinations were required involving multiple trips to Baltimore and each time one of my sisters would accompany me. The outpatient center at Johns Hopkins is the first building where international patients arrive. We were greeted in the International Lounge and seated with others from all over the world who were waiting to see the specialists. I had been assigned to an international coordinator who became the designated resource and communicator within the hospital. After that introduction, I greeted the financial advisor assigned to me who would be pre-approving all appointments and procedures while there.

Appointments with all surgeons were completed within the upper floors of the outpatient center. Once again, there was a process of checking in and ensuring that all documents were complete before the actual consultation. Then, the coordinator was required to escort international patients to each appointment. The neurosurgeon in Baltimore, whom others had recommended, was originally from Italy, and I was so thankful I had a sister in the room interpreting his strong foreign accent. I soon became confident in his abilities for success, but he himself warned me of the high risks involved in this particular surgery. This specialist was very personable and provided me with a direct phone number to call him if I had any questions or concerns before the expected surgery date.

I arrived back home from the first trip and started making plans. Knowing that there was a possibility the outcome of the surgery might be a dire one, I decided to ask more than one sibling to accompany me on the trip involving the actual surgery. Not because of the attention and time I might need for recuperation, but because if by chance of my passing, then that sibling would not be alone in a city far away from home.

Knowledge of the American medical system and how it differs from our Canadian one quickly became a necessity. In Canada, a patient is treated and as you are leaving, a facility administrator might request a discussion about the payment of extraneous costs. In the United States there are no examinations, treatments or interventions until it is confirmed who will be paying the total expenses. My second visit to Baltimore resulted in prolonged delays and interruptions to scheduled appointments because of the hospital's inability to understand or confirm that my provincial health plan would take care of the costs. A series of communications with the officials back in Regina who were approving this journey were needed while I sat for hours in Baltimore waiting for each appointment and medical test to be approved.

Before the actual surgery date, a new challenge needed to be resolved. Back home, I argued with officials that the province's restrictive process of approving payment each time a Band-aid (sarcasm) or X-ray was needed affected my chance of acquiring this surgery. The provincial officials were willing to write a letter to Johns Hopkins that gave open-ended permission of funding for the entire surgery process. This was precedent-setting for the province.

I then needed to convince personnel at Johns Hopkins Medicine, through telephone calls, that my English skills were substantial enough for me to traverse the hospital hallways on my own. I had assured them that I was able to transport my own financial permissions and hospital card without having to wait each time for a coordinator to accompany me. These successes were a time to celebrate and feel some degree of control within this entire journey.

The discussions with the officials of Saskatchewan Ministry of Health continued long after the actual procedure, including a face-to-face meeting with the Minister of Health a few months after my surgery. I felt that those influencing change needed to hear about the unique challenges of this particular medical journey and provided suggestions to create better processes for similar medical cases for other Little People in the future.

While my doctors and others assured me of the positive outcomes from this surgery, with an expected fifty per cent prediction of survival, my mind prior to the surgery was preparing for the worst. In preparation for travelling for this scheduled surgery, I had made sure that everything needed in my estate planning, including writing out funeral service arrangements, was completed just in case things did not go well. I wasn't depressed or wanting to die; I just wanted to be fully prepared and not leave anything tough for my family to address.

There were two buildings designated for surgeries at Johns Hopkins, and I was in the neurosurgical ward. When I woke up from surgery, I woke up surprised. I had expected to survive the surgery but after all the battles and stress of achieving this surgery I had little energy left for believing wonderful results would come from it. Allison even said that at times, right up to the actual surgery, I acted as if I was not going to wake up. I had a hard time believing this particularly hard journey was now complete.

I did wake up physically, but also seemed to wake up cognitively as well. I was being given a second chance and knew that I had to make sure I never forgot this opportunity because it was a gift.

A major surprise happened while in hospital when I first started to walk after surgery. The surgery had involved me having to lie face down for many hours during the procedure. The doctors put me in a coma-like effect for another twenty-four hours after the completion of the surgery to help reduce the swelling in my face, which was common after that type of surgery. I did not wake up until the next day and within six hours was out of bed walking up and down the hallways of the ward. I wasn't surprised I was walking so soon. I was surprised that I didn't have to think in order to walk.

What a concept! My entire life I had to think a certain way, talking to my legs to get them to move. The same with arm movement; I had always talked to my body when reaching for an item. I had no idea that walking could happen without conscious effort until those first few steps in that hospital hallway. I tried to explain repeatedly to my sisters this amazing change. What a gift it was to be able to walk without conscious effort!

My repeated visits to Baltimore, including my stay after surgery, provided time to get to know a city that is not as popular as other famous cities to Canadians touring the U.S.A. My sisters and I spent many hours admiring the marine views and spending time at the impressive National Aquarium. Baltimore is rich in history and impressive landmarks. The downtown area lies near the waterfront of Chesapeake Bay, with shopping and attractions surrounding one of the inlets.

To date, I have taken seven trips to the Johns Hopkins Hospital in Baltimore. The medical journey of my spine is a continual one and could fill another book in itself. My hope is that someday this particular medical journey, with others' words of wisdom regarding medical intervention, will be written for the benefit of other Little People and their medical professionals.

So what was I doing still alive? That is a question those LPA medical specialists asked and the same question I have sometimes asked of myself. The question of being alive is hard to answer since life is a perception only individuals can independently define.

At twenty-three years old, when writing the poem this book

is based on, I believed I was by no means normal, and I started questioning whether I wanted to continue being so abnormal. My siblings were fighting with each other. My friends were focussed on creating their own independence and new families. Strangers were treating me as either a celebrity or a freak. I was living in a town in southern Saskatchewan that was foreign to the customs and traditions I was used to. I felt very alone.

The quiet of living alone, the darkness of winter, the never-ending observance by strangers within this unknown community was too much. I wanted out. I wanted to be done. I made a vow, a promise to myself. I gave myself a deadline and told myself that I would keep to this deadline. Until my family, friends and even strangers have an opportunity to read this book, no one has been aware of the deadline I had given to myself.

On that particularly low day, so many years ago, I promised myself that if, in sixteen months on my twenty-fifth birthday, I was seeing my life in the same way as I was viewing it that day, I would not be having a twenty-sixth birthday. I scared myself with this promise, but knew that I could not go on viewing life without hope or a future. I never mentioned this promise to others; I did not reach out for medical help. I did not seek counsel or advice about this promise.

When I wrote the poem, I knew I had milestones to pass, but I had no idea what those milestones would be. Waiting sixteen months for my twenty-fifth birthday was the first milestone of my life. Realizing that the promise or pact I had made with myself was full of extreme emotion and not at all sane reassured me that I would never have carried out that promise.

Within six months of writing this poem, I chose, without any job prospects, to move back to my home community. My life continued and on my twenty-sixth birthday I did stop and reflect on the promise, or pact, I had made those two-and-a-half years before. Part of me was congratulating the wise decisions I had made since that time. Another part of me challenged me to keep on making wise decisions and moving forward in life.

Living through another fifteen years with the mistaken knowledge that the life expectancy of a Little Person was only to their forties was another milestone. I had lived life but continued to keep my true being distanced from others, believing I would die much earlier than my siblings, my friends and possibly even my parents. When I reached my early forties and discovered the falsehood of this information, it was only then that I started to live; I started to fight for me and realized that every challenge could be overcome. It has taken me another fifteen years to reach another milestone of finally sharing with others my life's lessons and expressing how important it is to welcome life through a variety of perspectives.

The title of this book was initially written in anger and frustration because of the never-ending misunderstandings people have of those who are different. However, like this writing, my life has evolved. The false perceptions were not of how people have viewed me, but how I had mistakenly viewed others and myself.

What is 'me' is understanding where I am going and where I am supposed to be. My being is from within and is always being portrayed on the surface. If I am comfortable and content with my presence, then that joy is reflected onto others. I know when I am whole and wanting to be within a particular space. I am one hundred per cent present and engaged with others. I am not thinking of my height difference or strategizing ways to accommodate myself into the present environment. I am just there. I leave each experience looking forward to the next time I can join that group or situation.

The future is open to possibilities and choices. I treasure relationships with family members who support independence and respect. I want to embrace my differences and help others overcome their fears about those whom they regard as different. I want to experience the kind of love I have witnessed repeatedly in family members and others. I want to explore and create new friendships while celebrating the ones I have been fortunate to maintain.

Who I was twenty years ago is not who I am today. Who I am today is not who I will be twenty years from now. This is what makes life so much fun. We really have limited control or power in predicting what our life will be like in the future. The only controls we have are the choices and decisions we can make today. Frequently, at the end of a piece of writing, whether it was a letter to a friend or a memo to staff members, I ended by writing, "Have a good day!" What you do today makes a difference to your tomorrows.

I have a role to play in this world, and it has nothing to do with my profession, my skills or my abilities. It is a role I have been participating in all my life and will continue to do for the rest of my years. It is my being, it is my existence, it is my true self and my need to share these perceptions with others.

The quest to be 'normal' will always be part of me

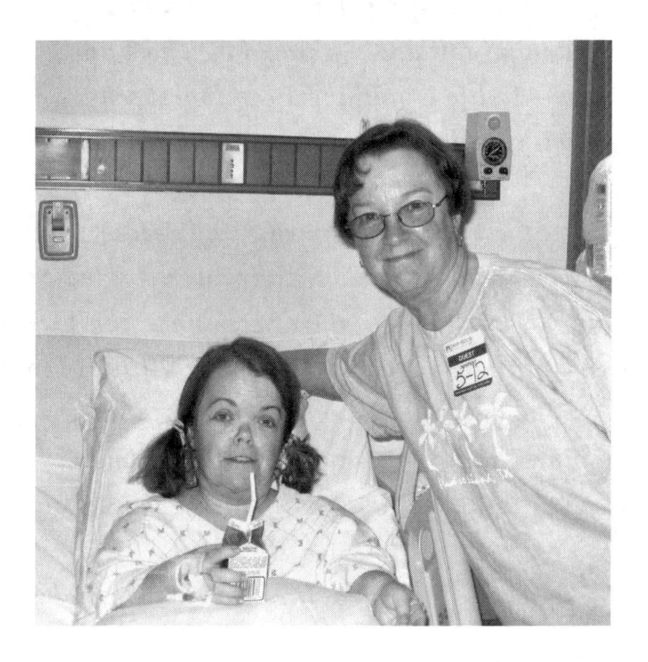

Allison and I in Baltimore.

Life is different because I am me.
I stand tall and am proud of who I am.
My life is full and I can look back
with pride, celebration, interest and joy.
The pride of my family,
their accomplishments and deeds.
The celebration of friends, their diversity and care.
The interest of strangers, their acceptance and journeys.
The joy of those I love, and the possibilities to come.
The gift of a kiss, of a dance, of a hug,
these things and more I can experience.
The quest to be 'normal' will always be part of me.

—L.J. Nelson, December 2016

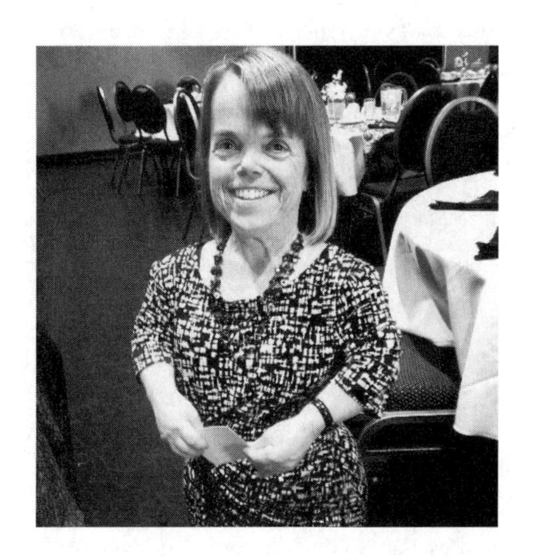

This is me.

Endnotes

1 LPA – Little People of America, Little People of America, Inc., 617 Broadway, #518 Sonoma, CA, U.S.A. 95476, www.lpaonline.org

2 Yehuda Koren and Eilat Negev. *In Our Hearts We Were Giants: The Remarkable Story of the Lilliput Troupe A Dwarf Family's Survival of the Holocaust*. (New York: Carroll & Graf Publishers, 2004).

3 *Marcus Welby, M.D.* (Television series: 1970–1975). Performed by Robert Young.

4 *Emergency!* (Television series: 1972–1977).
Performed by Randolph Mantooth and Kevin Tighe.

5 *M*A*S*H* (Television series: 1972–1983).* Performed by Alan Alda and Loretta Swit.

6 *Unconditional Love.* (Motion picture: 2003).Directed by P. J. Hogan. Performed by Kathy Bates and Rupert Everett.

[7] STF – Saskatchewan Teachers' Federation,
2317 Arlington Avenue, Saskatoon, SK, S7J 2H8

[8] Barr Colonists – www.esask.uregina.ca/entry/barr_colony.html

[9] Williamson, Marianne. *A Return to Love: Reflections on the Principles of "A Course in Miracles,"* Ch. 7, Section 3, 1992, 190.

[10] JHM – Johns Hopkins Medicine, 1800 Orleans Street, Baltimore, MD, U.S.A. 21287, www.hopkinsmedicine.org

[11] Greenburg Center for Skeletal Dysplasia, Johns Hopkins Hospital, 600 N. Wolfe Street, Baltimore, M.D., 21287,
www.hopkinsmedicine.org/institute-genetic-medicine/patient-care/genetics-clinic/about/greenberg-center-skeletal-dysplasia/

Acknowledgements

Thank you to FriesenPress. Your experience, knowledge and guidance in this self-publishing journey was greatly appreciated.

Thank you to Joan, Jessica and Marlene for your red-pen markings and sound advice.

Thank you to those friends and family members who were willing to read the rough passages and see the potential of my story.

L.J. Nelson

About the Author

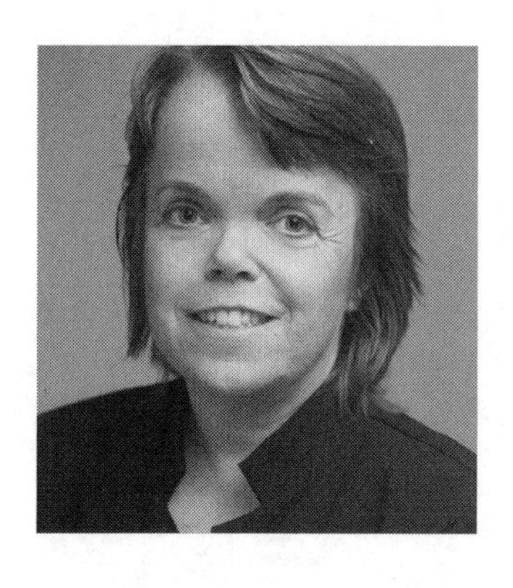

L.J. Nelson has been writing and storytelling for essentially all of her adult life. Her career as an educator has involved reams of technical writing for reports, policies, and guidelines. She has also written poetry and lyrics, and keeps various journals handy to record her thoughts and feelings. L.J.'s current role as a private tutor requires her to write monthly narratives about the lives of the students she works with. She sees herself as a storyteller who is learning to be a writer.

Printed in Canada